Frederick Stephens, AM, MD, FRCS (Ed), FACS, FRACS, is the Emeritus Professor of Surgery and Surgical Oncology and the former head of the Department of Surgery at the University of Sydney, and Consultant Surgeon Emeritus of Surgery and Surgical Oncology at the Royal Prince Alfred Hospital and Sydney Hospital.

Richard Fox, MB, BSc (med), PhD, FRACP, is the Director of Research at St Vincent's Hospital, the University of Melbourne, former Professor and Director of Clinical Haematology and Medical Oncology at the Royal Melbourne Hospital, and Vice President of the Cancer Council Victoria.

cancer
explained

THE ESSENTIAL GUIDE TO DIAGNOSIS AND MANAGEMENT

SECOND EDITION

Professor
FRED STEPHENS

Professor
RICHARD FOX

EBURY
PRESS

An Ebury Press book
Published by Random House Australia Pty Ltd
Level 3, 100 Pacific Highway, North Sydney, NSW 2060
www.randomhouse.com.au

First published by Wakefield Press in 1997
This second edition published by Ebury Press in 2008

Addresses for companies within the Random House Group can be found at www.randomhouse.com.au/offices.

National Library of Australia
Cataloguing-in-Publication Entry

Stephens, Fred, 1927–.
Cancer explained.

ISBN 978 1 74166 791 2 (pbk).

Cancer – Treatment – Popular works. Cancer – Treatment – Technological innovations. Cancer – Diagnosis.

Other authors/contributors: Fox, Richard.

616.994

Cover and internal image © Photolibrary
Cover and internal design by Melanie Fedderson/www.i2i.com.au
Typeset in 10.5/16 pt Minion by Midland Typesetters, Australia
Printed and bound by Griffin Press, South Australia

Random House Australia uses papers that are natural, renewable and recyclable products and made from wood grown in sustainable forests. The logging and manufacturing processes are expected to conform to the environmental regulations of the country of origin.

10 9 8 7 6 5 4 3 2 1

contents

Section 4: Where do we go from here? 233

foreword to first edition

At long last we have a comprehensive, readable and understandable book on cancer, a book that does not scare but puts the entire topic in its true perspective. *Cancer Explained* helps remove much of the mystique, horror and hopelessness that many people associate with cancer. This book is filled with page after page of good cheer, as we see countless ways in which everyone can take steps – usually simple ones – to help prevent the disease from striking. That is marvellous news in itself. Although most of these steps have been known for years, they are brought together in *Cancer Explained* in an easily followed way. Then we are gently walked through the various forms of cancer, the signs and symptoms which should alert us and the steps the doctor will take in diagnosis and treatment. Finally there are simple explanations of the litany of cancer-related words.

Cancer Explained is filled with common sense, empathy and hard-hitting facts, all wrapped up in words that anyone can follow and understand. Western medicine still offers the most important options in dealing with cancer. But the book shows an appreciation of the enormous range of 'alternative' methods of prevention and treatment. Many accepted forms of Western medicine are based on naturally occurring products. Fred

Stephens acknowledges the proliferating data on fibre, isoflavi-noids and phytoestrogens, and their value in prevention – a reason why cancer is so rare in countries where legumes and other high-fibre, low-fat foods are part of the everyday diet. There are lessons to be learned from all parts of the globe.

Fred Stephens has a long and distinguished association with cancer and education, at the University of Sydney, Sydney Hospital and the Royal Prince Alfred Hospital. For many years he educated, advised and treated vast numbers of students and patients. All have benefited from his experience and, just as importantly, from his understanding and empathy for his fellow human beings.

I am intrigued by this fine book and recommend it to medical people as well as everyone out there. Reading it will help you better understand all aspects of the second-largest killer in our community. And it will help you save lives, most importantly your own, or that of family or friends.

Read this book, and tell your friends to read it also. I am certainly recommending it to my media audience.

Dr James Wright, AM, MB, BS, FRACGP

foreword to second edition

Cancer control is a fast-moving field, and it is pleasing that this useful cancer reference book for the general public has been updated. The changes reflect our better understanding of this common and misunderstood disease, and the advances in diagnosis and treatment that have occurred over the last decade.

Books cannot take the place of personal discussions with a healthcare team, nor can they cover all aspects of cancer control in depth. However, this book will help the general public, particularly the cancer patient and his or her family, to understand the issues and the words that they will come across in the course of the cancer journey. Cancer is increasingly a preventable and curable disease, and a cancer diagnosis should no longer be the cause of fear that it once was. Knowledge helps dispel fear, and this book will assist people in asking the questions to which they need answers.

Professor Ian Frazer, MB, ChB (Ed), MD (Melbourne), FRCPA, MRCP, Australian of the Year, 2006

comments of the former Chairman of the NSW Cancer Council

Surgical oncologist Professor Fred Stephens and medical oncologist Professor Richard Fox have provided one of the best and most comprehensive guides to all aspects of cancer for anyone with an interest and involvement in this now very common medical problem. *Cancer Explained* covers all the general information needed to understand how cancer develops, why it is sometimes able to spread within the body and become fatal, and how it is managed and most often cured. For those with a specific cancer problem the second half of the book provides detailed information on the diagnosis and management of most common cancers.

Written in an easy-to-read style, the book provides an essential overview of current information on cancer and a valuable reference for those who develop cancer. The authors stress the curability of most cancers with modern multidisciplinary management and provide valuable advice on prevention, early diagnosis and current therapies.

The second edition expands and brings up to date what was, in the first edition, a comprehensive source of information on cancer for the general community.

Emeritus Professor William McCarthy, AM, MB,
BS (Sydney), M Ed (Illinois)

preface to first edition

My intention in writing this book has been to answer the questions that patients and friends ask me about cancer. It is intended to help not only cancer patients, or friends and family of cancer patients, but also nurses and paramedical personnel. The book should also help medical practitioners to answer patients' questions and perhaps give them a broader understanding of the various aspects of cancer.

Section 1 will be of interest to all people concerned about cancer. It describes what cancer means, what is known about its causes, who is at risk and how it might be prevented.

Section 2 describes the general and local features of cancer, test procedures, special investigations that might be helpful and what the patient might expect in having these investigations carried out. It also outlines the different forms of treatment that are available.

Section 3 deals with specific types of cancer in different parts of the body. Readers may wish to read only that part which is of particular concern to them.

Section 4 is a short review of possible new challenges and likely advances in cancer treatment in the future.

A glossary and an index provide, respectively, definitions of all medical terminology used and a cross-reference to all sections.

I hope that this book will not only give the lay reader a better understanding of the problems of cancer but also help all who care for people with cancer. It is only by promoting a better understanding of the clinical realities and the therapeutic possibilities of cancer that the social and emotional needs of patients and those who love and care for them will be met.

Professor Fred Stephens

preface to second edition

This second edition of *Cancer Explained* updates the original version written ten years ago. It explains the present understanding, features, investigations, treatments and likely outcomes in cancer treatment today and describes significant advances both in current practice and practices under study. For anything but the most simple and uncomplicated cancers, cancer doctors now need to work in multidisciplinary teams often specialising in only one or two tumour types. This allows them to develop and maintain the sophisticated skills needed for today's therapies as well as future roles in cancer care.

The authors wish to acknowledge the inspiration given to them by the dedicated work of many colleagues and friends in the medical and nursing professions as well as the research, secretarial and administrative fields, both in Australia and overseas. Many of these people have been the unsung contributors to current success stories in the care of people with cancer. Such exciting advances include the change in outlook for patients with melanoma: in our student days it was a disease with about a 50% mortality rate. Now this is less than 10% in Australian clinics.

Similarly the outlooks for acute leukaemia in children, acute myeloid leukaemia in adults, advanced testicular cancer in young men, chorionic carcinoma in women of child-bearing age, Hodgkin (also known as Hodgkin's) and other lymphomas in young adults have all changed. From being considered virtually incurable, these have become almost always curable cancers.

Most once-standard mutilating surgical procedures, such as amputation of a limb, total removal of a breast or radical surgery to the head and neck, can now be avoided by multi-modality management in combined specialist clinics, with at least equally satisfactory curative results. This reflects the integration of minimalist surgery with radiotherapy and chemotherapy.

Anti-smoking campaigns and other public-health measures have resulted in reduced numbers of people dying from smoking- and asbestos-related cancers.

Early detection measures have resulted in reduced numbers dying from advanced breast cancer, cervical cancer, bowel cancer, prostate cancer and stomach cancer.

Preventive measures are now well established for many cancers, and this information is readily available to individuals, families and their communities. Cancer of the cervix in women will shortly be a largely preventable disease, thanks to the work of 2005 Australian of the Year Professor Ian Frazer in developing preventive vaccines.

Integrated treatment centres, more effective anti-cancer drugs, targeted biologics, more effective radiotherapeutic procedures and remarkable improvements in plastic and recon-structive surgery have all improved the outlook for most individuals and the community at large.

Finally, for those not as yet able to be cured, improvements in palliative care are now more readily available to make their lives more worthwhile and more comfortable.

Professor Fred Stephens and Professor Richard Fox

1

questions
commonly
asked about
cancer

WHAT IS CANCER?

The word 'cancer' is a Latin word meaning 'crab'. The condition was called cancer in ancient times because an advanced cancer was thought to resemble a crab with claws reaching out into surrounding tissues. A cancer, or malignant growth, is now known to be a continuous, purposeless, unwanted, uncontrolled and damaging growth of cells. Cancers are also referred to as 'tumours', but this word just means a lump, so it can also refer to non-malignant growths.

Although most normal body tissues contain cells that have the ability to grow or reproduce, they do so only when there is a need; when the need has been satisfied, the growth stops. For example, cells in some tissues such as the skin or blood wear out quickly and are constantly being replaced. Cells reproduce only to meet the immediate needs of the body. However, in the case of a cancer, cell reproduction continues for no good reason, and excessive numbers of abnormal cells are produced; there is no 'switching off' mechanism. The abnormal and unwanted cells spread into surrounding tissues, causing damage. The abnormal cancer cells also tend to invade blood and lymph vessels, where they may travel to other parts of the body and establish new colonies of growing cells. These colonies are called secondary (or 'metastatic') cancers.

A cancer is quite different from an infection. An infection is caused when germs or organisms from outside the body invade body tissues, causing damage. The body's defences recognise the germs as foreign material and establish protective measures to destroy these invading organisms. Invading cancer cells, on the other hand, are abnormal cells that have developed from the body's own cells. They are, consequently, often not recognised by the body's defences as being foreign and tend to grow and invade without being attacked by this defence mechanism.

A growth of cells that seems to be under some sort of control is called a benign tumour. Although there is no apparent purpose in the growth, the cells are more mature and closely resemble the cells of the tissue from which they developed. Once the growth reaches a certain size, it usually slows down or stops growing any further. All the cells of a benign tumour stay together as a lump or swelling that is usually confined by a capsule, or lining of fibrous tissue made from the adjoining tissue. They do not spread to other parts of the body.

With cancer, or malignant growth, on the other hand, the cells look abnormal and less like the cells from which they developed. As a rule, the more malignant the tumour the more abnormal the cells appear. The multiplication of cells also continues without control, causing the tumour to get bigger and bigger. The tumour may then invade surrounding body tissues, increasing the likelihood of it spreading to other parts of the body and establishing secondary growths.

Types of cancer

Although all malignant growths are commonly referred to as cancers, the word 'cancer' (or 'carcinoma') is more correctly applied to a malignant growth of glandular cells, cells lining a hollow organ or a duct, or cells lining skin surfaces. Cancers of the flat cells lining the skin and some hollow organs such as the oesophagus (gullet), mouth or throat are called squamous carcinomas, and cancers of gland cells (more round, ball shaped, or rectangular/brick shaped) are called adenocarcinomas. A cancer may start in cells lining the mouth, throat, stomach or bowel, cells lining the ducts of the breast or cells lining the air passages in the lungs, cells lining the cavity of the uterus or vagina, the kidney or bladder. A cancer may start in any organ where there are glandular structures, such as the thyroid gland, the prostate gland, glandular tissue of the breast, the pancreas, the salivary glands and the liver or the kidneys.

Malignant tumours of these glands or lining cells are truly called cancers and are the most common forms of malignant tumour. However, sometimes cells of other tissues (such as blood, bone, the brain or muscle) will become malignant (i.e. grow continuously, without purpose and without control or restraint). Although these are commonly called cancers, they are more correctly called by other names, as described in Section 3 of this book.

ARE ALL TUMOURS MALIGNANT?

The answer is 'no'. Non-malignant or benign tumours are, in general, much more common than malignant tumours.

IS CANCER ALWAYS DANGEROUS?

If a cancer is detected early, if it is small and has not yet spread to other parts of the body, it can usually be removed surgically or treated – with radiotherapy and/or chemotherapy – so that it is cured.

Cancers are dangerous when they cause damage and destruction to surrounding tissues and when they spread to other organs and tissues where they establish secondary cancers (metastases). These secondary growths damage and interfere with the function of the organ or tissue in which they are growing. For example, secondary cancers in the liver interfere with the function of the liver. If secondaries are in the lung, they can block air passages and interfere with breathing, causing infection or pneumonia. Secondaries in the brain will cause pressure on the brain and interfere with its function, and secondaries in bones can cause pain and erosion of bone, which may then collapse or fracture.

Most skin cancers (including melanoma) are now detected when they are small and easily cured. However, it is now recognised that with modern treatment and early diagnosis, some 55% of all of the more serious internal cancers in patients in developed countries can be cured. If lung cancer was taken out of the equation – by people stopping smoking – then the cure rates overall would be well over 60%.

HOW COMMON IS CANCER?

Cancer is known to occur in all societies and in all parts of the world. It affects animals as well as humans. Cancer occurred in ancient as well as in modern times. However, the types of cancer most prevalent in a community vary with the age, sex and race of those in the community, as well as its geographical location. These various forms of cancer will reflect the economic and environmental conditions of the different countries, and in particular their diet and lifestyle.

In Westernised societies cancer is responsible for about 25% of deaths. As lifespan progressively lengthens, cancer is becoming a more significant cause of death than heart and vascular disease. The most common cancers in Western developed countries are those of the prostate, breast, lung and colorectum (large bowel). These account for more than half the known cancer cases, other than the common skin cancers.

The relationship between these cancers and age is striking. Most people are surprised to know that from the age of 50 to 59 there is a one in 20 chance that an individual will develop a cancer (excluding a simple skin cancer). To go from 60 to 69 the chance is one in ten and from 70 to 79 one in five. Once individuals get over the age of 80, there is a one in three chance that they will develop a cancer.

Young people in Western society, meanwhile, are more at risk from accidents at home or on the road, because cancer is relatively uncommon in this age group. The rarer cancers in young people are usually of a quite different type: leukaemias (cancers of the blood cells), lymphomas (cancers of the bone marrow and lymph nodes), certain sarcomas (bone or soft-tissue cancers) and testicular cancer in males.

WHAT CAUSES CANCER?

For generations doctors, researchers, philosophers and quacks have been trying to find a single cause for all cancers and consequently a single cure. This is unlikely because cancers are the result of many different causes.

Cancer begins when one or more of the trillions of cells in

our bodies breaks free of normal restraints and starts to divide and multiply in an uncontrolled way. This can happen to almost any kind of cell, especially those cells that frequently divide to replace worn-out cells, such as skin, glands, stomach- or bowel-lining cells and blood-forming cells.

Cancers are many different diseases and can occur in virtually every organ. There are quite different causes for these various cancers. Like all animals and plants we inherit two sets of genes, one from each of our parents. Genes are chains of DNA (deoxyribonucleic acid) with specific coding sequences in the nucleus of cells. Genes are responsible for transmitting inherited features from our parents. Genes determine the colour of our skin and eyes, our height and other obvious body features but also the many different tissues, organs and cells in the total make-up of our bodies and body functions. Genes are in two sets of small chains called chromosomes in each cell nucleus. They are also responsible for cell division and needed for tissue growth and repair. A cancer is formed when there has been a change in one or more genes (mutation) so that new cells are produced when they are not needed.

Normal cell division is under the control of genes in the nucleus. There are many different factors that can trigger mutations in the genes (DNA) of cells. It now appears that to form cancer cells a sequence of several genes in the DNA is mutated. This process may take many years to occur. These mutations alter the balance of control of cell division or replication. Other types of genes cause cells to die as a normal process (e.g. those lining the bowel or lung airways). Loss of activity of these genes due to mutation may lead to cells with a long lifespan, creating abnormal growth. Other genes in the cancer cell are responsible for tissue invasion and the ability to travel in the blood or lymph streams and seed elsewhere, rather like the seeds of weeds caught in the wind and spreading in a garden.

Most recent studies suggest that many cancers may result from a combination of these factors. Cells contain genes (specific DNA sequences) that 'switch on' a self-limiting repair process when a tissue is worn out or injured. After repair the healing mechanism is 'switched off' by other genes. Cancer-causing agents, such as certain viruses, chemicals or, most commonly, random mutations, may accumulate with age, causing abnormal cell reproduction. Many of these mutated genes are called oncogenes and produce abnormal signal proteins that trigger the switch-on mechanism for cell replication. There is evidence that some people inherit abnormal oncogenes in their genomes, predisposing them to a greater risk of developing cancer.

It is now recognised that in a small proportion of patients with cancers – particularly breast, bowel and ovarian cancer – the oncogenes may be transmitted through families. Individuals in such families are at greater risk for the development of these cancers.

There is a wide range of potential causes of the various cancers, although in many individuals a specific cause may not be identified. Tobacco smoking is a major cause and is responsible for an increased incidence of cancers of the lung, mouth, throat and larynx, as well as cancers of the oesophagus, stomach, pancreas, kidney, bladder and even the breast.

Excessive exposure to ultraviolet light from the sun is responsible for an increased incidence of skin cancers in fair-skinned people who live in regions closer to the equator. Reflecting this, Australia has the highest incidence of skin cancers in the world. Certain lifestyle factors appear to be related to the development of colorectal, prostate and breast cancer. These include a Western-style diet (high animal fat, low fibre) as well as a more sedentary lifestyle.

Some industrial irritants and chemical carcinogens (cancer-causing substances) cause different types of cancers. The first cancer found in Western countries to be caused by a chemical agent was cancer of the scrotum, which commonly developed in chimney sweeps in Britain in the eighteenth century. The cause was found to be soot, which collected in the scrotal area of those industrial workers. Later, certain dyes used by German workers in chemical factories and excreted in the urine were found to be associated with an increased incidence of bladder cancer. People using phosphorus to paint luminous dials on clocks and watches were also found to have a high incidence of bone cancer. The phosphorus was absorbed due to the workers' habit of licking the tips of their small phosphorus paintbrushes. These types of cancer are not seen today because of improved working conditions. A number of chemical agents cause cancer in exper-imental animals. Similar agents are present in tobacco tars and products of the petroleum industry and other chemical industries. Asbestos exposure is associated with the development of malignant mesothelioma, a quite rare cancer of the lining of the lung or the abdominal cavity.

Viruses have been studied as a possible cause for human cancer, based on evidence that certain ones cause cancers in animals and that, in humans, warts are known to be caused by a virus. (A wart is a benign tumour.) However, apart from a few exceptions, there is no clear evidence that common viruses are responsible for cancer in humans.

The exceptions include a certain cancer in the back of the nose and upper throat, most common in Chinese people who live in or near the Guangdong province of China near Hong Kong. In these people there is a high incidence of infection with the Epstein-Barr virus, which may play a part in developing this cancer. The Epstein-Barr virus, which is associated with infectious mononucleosis (glandular fever), may also be linked to the development of some lymphomas, especially a highly malignant form of lymphoma described as Burkitt's lymphoma, which occurs in children, particularly in Africa and New Guinea.

A virus responsible for hepatitis C is a risk factor for the development of hepatocellular carcinoma (hepatoma), a primary liver cancer. This is a common cancer in South East Asia.

The human papilloma virus is responsible for the development of cancer of the entrance of the uterus (cervical cancer), as well as cancer of the penis. The virus is commonly transmitted sexually.

Although rarely seen today, people with AIDS (acquired immune deficiency syndrome) were at greater risk for Kaposi's sarcoma, which was a malignant transformation of small blood vessels in the skin and gastrointestinal tract.

In India and New Guinea, where betel-nut or tobacco leaf is chewed, there is a dramatic increase in the incidence of cancer of the mouth and pharynx. This appears to be due to a direct carcinogenic effect of the betel-nut or tobacco leaf on the lining cells of the mouth.

However, for the majority of individuals with a cancer there is often no known cause, apart from age, Western lifestyle and diet. For instance, approximately 100 years ago cancer of the stomach (gastric cancer) was much more common than it is today. Since the introduction of both commercial and domestic refrigeration with improved food-handling habits and less use of preservatives in food, the incidence of gastric cancer has gone down significantly. An exception to this is in Japan and some eastern countries where there are different food habits and a different diet. By comparison, the risk for bowel cancer has gone up with the modern Western diet.

It is also a common observation that pre-existing abnormalities in tissue are more likely to develop malignant cells than normal tissues. Such abnormal tissues include congenitally abnormal tissues, chronically irritated tissues, chronically wasted or worn out (atrophic) tissues, chronically inflamed or severely scarred tissues or tissues with one or more surface sores (ulcers). Pre-existing benign tumours such as lumps under the surface lining of the skin or mouth, or lumps projecting from such a surface (polyps or papillomas), also have an increased chance of malignant change.

WHO IS AT RISK?

The single greatest factor for the risk of developing cancer is age, as described earlier. The other major risk factors are smoking and certain aspects of Western living, including diet and a sedentary lifestyle. These are also risk factors for cardiovascular disease and diabetes. Excessive sun exposure, particularly for leisure activities, is an obvious risk factor for skin cancers, including melanoma.

A family history of cancer (particularly in breast or bowel if it has developed in family members by their 40s and 50s) may indicate an increased risk in that family, possibly due to an inherited oncogene.

Individuals who have had treatment for a particular cancer, which may have included radiation therapy and/or prolonged chemotherapy, may be at increased risk for the development of a second cancer. For example, smokers who have developed cancer of the oral cavity, which may be cured by treatment, are at high risk for the development of lung cancer if they continue to smoke.

As people grow older the risk of something going wrong with the cell-division process over its many generations is increased, so that genetic mutations are more likely to cause development of abnormal, cancerous cells.

IS CANCER CONTAGIOUS?

No. There is no evidence that, in the normal course of events, cancer can be passed from one individual to another. However, there are certain viral infections that lead to organ damage that can subsequently lead to cancer. For instance, primary cancer of the liver (hepatoma), which is a common disease in Asia, may be a sequel to a chronic infection with the hepatitis B or hepatitis C virus causing cirrhosis. The hepatitis virus can spread if there is poor personal hygiene and faecal contamination.

Similarly cancer of the cervix (neck of womb) is often a sequel of genital infection with the human papilloma virus. This virus is spread by sexual contact. A small proportion of women infected with this virus will go on to develop cancer of the cervix and, much more rarely, men will develop cancer of the penis.

Prior to the development of effective antiviral therapy, AIDS, which is caused by viral infection (HIV 1), may have predisposed people to certain cancers. These include malignant lymphoma and Kaposi's sarcoma, which is a malignancy of small blood vessels in the skin and gastrointestinal tract. The cause of malignancy in patients with AIDS is the damage to the patient's natural immune defences against both infection and cancer. Even though a number of individuals still have AIDS, much of the immune deficit is controlled by antiviral therapy, and the risk of developing these cancers is much less. Sadly, though, this antiviral therapy is only readily available in Western countries.

DOES HEREDITY PLAY A PART?

It is now known that perhaps some 5–10% of cancers are due to mutations, that is changes in cancer-susceptibility genes that are inherited. There are some well-recognised risk factors that may indicate a genetic cancer syndrome is present in a family. One is that the cancer has come on at a relatively early age (e.g. under the age of 45 for breast cancer or under the age of 50 for a patient with bowel cancer or prostate cancer).

Other indicative factors are the presence of several family members on the same side of a family with a similar cancer. A cluster of various cancers is known to stem from a single gene change. Thus any combination of breast, ovarian, uterine or bowel cancer in two or more members of a family often indicates genetic influence. Another factor would be where one individual has multiple, or a series of, primary cancers (e.g. both breast and ovarian cancer, or multiple primary cancers of the large bowel).

There are now, in special hospital centres, family-counselling clinics that can assist patients and their families in understanding the potential risks for the development of cancer in other family members. There are also sophisticated gene tests (DNA typing) for a variety of these hereditary cancers. These tests, which can be done only in specialised centres, are expensive and the technical process is quite complex and often takes several months to carry out. The more commonly known genetic mutations are in breast cancer, due to genes called BCRA 1 and BCRA 2, and in colon cancer due to genes called APC and MMR.

Family members may need to be followed up with screening examinations if they are at high risk. Issues of confidentiality and privacy are carefully attended to in these clinics.

DOES AGE PLAY A PART?

As discussed earlier, the risk of developing most cancers increases progressively with age. However, although it is relatively rare, cancer can occur in infancy, young children and teenagers. The types of cancers that occur at these young ages are quite different from those occurring in adults. They are often called 'blastic' or 'blastomas' because they arise from immature 'blast' cells. Such cancers include acute lymphoblastic leukaemia and Wilms' tumour (nephroblastoma), which is a type of cancer of the kidney. When the latter does occur, it is almost always in infants less than five years of age and may even be present at birth. Treatment is surgery and chemotherapy. The survival rate for most of the children with this tumour is now really quite good with modern treatment.

Another childhood cancer is neuroblastoma, arising from nerve cells, which occurs generally in the abdominal cavity. Children are treated with surgery and chemotherapy. Depending on the extent of the disease and the nature of the particular cancer, most children with early-stage disease have very good outcomes following surgery. Another rare cancer is called rhab-domyosarcoma, which is a malignancy of muscle tissue in infants and children.

Teenagers and young adults can develop acute leukaemias and lymphomas. These are cancers of blood cells and lymph nodes and include Hodgkin lymphoma. The outlook for many with these lymphomas is extremely good with modern radiotherapy and chemotherapy. Burkitt's lymphoma is a cancer that predominantly affects the jaws of children, most commonly in tropical Africa and New Guinea (see the discussion of viruses in 'What causes cancer?' earlier).

Teenagers and young adults have the highest incidence of bone cancers. Bone cancers (osteosarcomas) are relatively uncommon, but when they do occur it is most often during the growth periods of children and young adults.

Malignant tumours of the testes are quite rare but occur most commonly in men between the ages of 20 and 40. Again, with appropriate surgery and chemotherapy, the cure rates are extremely high. The best known example of this good outcome is the champion Tour de France cyclist Lance Armstrong. He had advanced testicular cancer cured with modern chemotherapy and surgery.

Ovarian cancer and cancer of the cervix most commonly affect women between the ages of 40 and 60, but cancer of the body of the uterus is more likely to occur in women over the age of 60.

The common cancers of the lung, prostate, bowel and breast all occur more frequently in older people, particularly over the age of 50, increasing in incidence with age, as discussed earlier. Lung cancer has become increasingly common in communities where cigarette smoking is prevalent. The average age at onset is about 70, as it takes many years for the irritating effects of tobacco tars to cause the changes in the air passages that lead to cancer. However, tragically, individuals who commence smoking as teenagers may develop the disease in their late 30s or 40s.

Breast cancer is uncommon in women under 30 years. Thereafter it increases in incidence with age, having a median age of onset of about 60 years.

The incidence of stomach and bowel cancers also increases with age, reaching a peak incidence at about 70 years of age.

Cancer of the prostate gland is another disease of increasing age. It is not often seen in men under 50 but is the most common internal cancer affecting men over 65, and some slowly developing, apparently malignant cells can be seen in the prostate gland of virtually all men over the age of 90.

Skin cancers and oropharyngeal (mouth and throat) cancers become more common with increasing age. The cause of most skin cancers is cumulative damage to skin, which may reflect outdoor exposure since childhood and sunburns. Similarly, melanoma is related to skin damage caused by sun exposure. Although it is rare before puberty, after puberty it occurs in people of all age groups, gradually becoming more common with increasing age. Unlike other skin cancers, which most often occur on the face because that skin is most constantly exposed to the sun, melanoma is not so directly related to gradual prolonged sunlight exposure. Melanoma occurs most commonly on the parts of the body and lower limbs that are not constantly exposed to the sun but are more likely to have been damaged by occasional episodes of sunburn. This presumably reflects recreational exposure, often as a child.

ARE SOME PEOPLE MORE LIKELY TO DEVELOP CANCER THAN OTHERS?

Clearly the answer to this is 'yes'. There are several so-called pre-malignant conditions that can lead to the development of malignant change and hence cancer. Although most cancers develop 'out of the blue' in tissues that were apparently otherwise normal, many cancers develop in tissues that have been chronically damaged. Abnormal tissues are more likely to develop malignant change.

The most common of these is repeated sun damage to skin. Apart from the wrinkling and thickening of the skin, there may be small discrete areas where the skin is thickened and crusty, called hyperkeratoses. This is a pre-malignant condition, and within these small hyperkeratotic areas a skin cancer termed a squamous-cell carcinoma may develop. These are particularly common on the face, lips and backs of hand. Malignant melanoma may develop in a pre-existing, apparently benign mole or a pigmented naevus, although sometimes melanoma develops in an apparently normal area of skin with no evidence of a pre-existing mole.

People who have pernicious anaemia (a blood disorder) or chronic atrophic gastritis (a stomach disorder) have a six-times greater risk of developing stomach cancer than other people.

Stomach ulcers too may occasionally develop into stomach cancers, although the more common duodenal ulcer has not shown any tendency to develop into cancer.

Another important pre-malignant condition is the presence of benign adenomas or polyps in the large bowel (colon or rectum). These can, over the years, undergo a malignant change. Individuals may be detected with these because of investigation for rectal bleeding. The polyps are usually removed by simple resection using an endoscope (an instrument for examining the interior of the bowel).

Chronic inflammatory conditions of the bowel, such as ulcerative colitis and granular colitis (Crohn's disease), can also lead to the development of cancer of the large bowel. Ulcerative colitis has a much greater tendency to do this, and the risk of cancer is related to the extent and duration of ulcerative colitis in the bowel lining. Because of this risk, many individuals with ulcerative colitis may have their large bowel totally or partially surgically removed. The younger the patient at the onset of ulcerative colitis, the longer it has been present, and the greater the extent of the colitis in the colon, the greater the risk of cancer developing.

Smokers are particularly prone to developing chronic irritation of the mucosal lining of the mouth and throat. This may lead to a thickening of the surface cell layer that shows up as small white patches (leukoplakia). These patches also have a predisposition towards the development of a subsequent cancer (squamous-cell carcinoma).

Chronic inflammatory conditions involving the gall bladder, kidney and bladder associated with stones can predispose these organs to the subsequent development of cancer.

Although relatively rare today, chronic leg ulcers associated with either repeated trauma or unhealed varicose ulcers can sometimes develop into the so-called Marjolin's cancer involving the skin area around the ulcer. This is more common as a sequel to longstanding chronic tropical ulcers involving the leg.

Women who have chronic mastitis in the breasts (more correctly known as benign mammary dysplasia, hormonal mastopathy or fibroadenosis cystica) have a slightly higher risk of developing breast cancer.

Rarely, a benign tumour may become malignant. With some types of benign tumours such as warts, the risk is extremely small, virtually negligible. With the common fatty tumour called a lipoma, the risk is so small that removal is usually not justified. However, with others there is a small but somewhat greater risk of malignant change, and for many of them surgical removal of the lump is usually recommended. These include papilloma (a fern-like projecting tumour) in the mouth or in a duct of a breast or sometimes colon; some soft-tissue tumours (tumours of fat, fibrous tissue, nerves, blood vessels, etc.); adenomas (gland lumps); and benign tumours of bone or cartilage. With still other benign tumours, such as polyps of the stomach or colon or especially papilloma of the rectum, the risk of malignant change is of real significance and surgical removal of these tumours is virtually always recommended.

Certain congenital abnormalities can subsequently undergo a malignant change. These include a thyroglossal cyst (a congenital remnant of thyroid tissue high in the neck or in the back of the tongue) and a branchial cyst (a cyst resulting from a congenital developmental abnormality in the neck). Another important abnormality is an undescended testis, where the testis has not descended into the scrotum at birth but remains at the back of the abdominal cavity. This has an increased risk of developing cancer. This is important as surgeons can bring the testis down into the scrotum or remove it. These increased risks are of varying degrees. The risk is very small in the case of branchial cysts but quite high in the case of an undescended testis.

Lipomas, which are common benign fatty tumours often underneath the skin, very rarely develop a malignant change, but internal lipomas are more likely to undergo a malignant change, becoming a sarcoma. It is also important to note that there does not appear to be any significant risk of the development of a tumour (sarcomas in bone or muscle) after acute injuries such as a kick in the thigh or a blow to a bone at football, etc. However, some individuals with these tumours do report a preceding injury. This is much more likely to have drawn attention to a pre-existing sarcoma rather than caused it.

DOES GENDER PLAY A PART?

Obviously, cancers that occur in organs of one sex only are unique to that sex. Surprisingly, breast cancer can occur in men.

However, for every 100 cases that occur in women, there is only one occurring in men. The treatment and outcome is virtually the same in men as it is in women.

Lung cancer was once predominantly a male-related disease, reflecting the predominance of cigarette smoking in men. The incidence of lung cancer has increased since World War II. However, the incidence in women is rising dramatically, particularly in the United States, and is approaching the levels seen in men. This reflects the increase in smoking by women. It is of considerable concern that there is a high level of smoking in teenage girls, which is anticipated to cause a further increase in the incidence of lung cancer in women in a few decades.

Generally skin cancers are more common in men because of the increased exposure to the sun in recreational activities and outdoor work. This usually reflects sun exposure some decades earlier, when there was little awareness of skin protection, when block-out creams were not used and people spent significant time outdoors without a hat or shirt.

Stomach cancer is two or three times more likely to occur in men than in women in most countries but not all, possibly reflecting the relative incidence of smoking in some communities.

There are also some slight differences in gender incidence in some other cancers for no apparent reason. For example, cancer of the oesophagus is more common in men, especially in the middle and lower oesophagus, but cancer in the upper oesophagus is more common in women. Also, for unknown reasons, cancer of the rectum is more common in men, but cancer of the colon is slightly more common in women.

Primary carcinoma of the liver (hepatoma) is some three-fold higher in males, probably because of greater alcohol consumption. The incidence of cancer of the pancreas, more common in men, is increasing in the USA, especially in men who are smokers. It is also being seen more frequently in women with diabetes mellitus and women smokers.

DOES DIET PLAY A PART?

The predominant dietary issue is the role of fat consumption as a cancer risk. International differences in the incidence of several cancers have been correlated with apparent per-capita fat consumption. The strongest associations have been seen with cancer of the breast, colon, prostate and lining of the womb (endometrium). These are the most common internal cancers in the Western world, with the exception of lung cancer, which is essentially smoking induced. Therefore, reduction in dietary fat has been important in cancer prevention strategies.

Fat and breast cancer

While breast cancer is the most common cancer in women in Western countries, the association between fat and breast cancer is complex and controversial. It may be that the relatively lower incidence in Mediterranean countries reflects the use of mono-unsaturated fats (olive oil as distinct from animal fats). It may also be that animal fats, including human fat, store various hormones that may increase the risk of breast cancer.

In the West the age of puberty has been dropping for many years. It may be that high overall energy/food consumption allows rapid growth rates and leads to early puberty, with increased years of menstrual cycles producing oestrogen (female sex hormone) over a more prolonged fertile lifespan. This may play a role in the future risk of development of breast cancer.

Fat and bowel cancer

Apart from dietary fibre it is not entirely clear whether the higher rates of colorectal cancer in affluent Western countries most reflect increased fat intake or an association with a sedentary lifestyle. There is some association between total energy (food) intake and bowel cancer but not with the amounts of various fats.

Studies in Australia suggest that the consumption of processed meats increases the risk of cancer of the rectum.

Fat and prostate cancer

There is some relationship between prostate-cancer mortality and consumption of animal fat.

In general people who wish to reduce their risk of cancer are advised to reduce their intake of foods high in animal fat. This is also a sound recommendation for reducing the risk of cardio-vascular disease.

A general health recommendation is to have a balanced diet coupled with adequate physical activity.

It is interesting to note that 100 years ago in the Western world cancer of the stomach was one of the most common cancers. Its incidence has dramatically decreased. This appears to correlate with the introduction of commercial and domestic refrigeration. This may mean that in Western countries meat is fresher and less likely to be contaminated with micro-organisms. There is also less reliance on various curing processes involving salts, other chemicals, smoking of food, etc. It is thought that some of these processes led to a high incidence of gastric cancer at that time.

Fibre and bowel cancer

The potential role of fibre in the diet in relation to cancer has been intensively studied. Most studies have indicated that a high-fibre diet appears to be protective against bowel cancer. Whether this is a mechanical effect of the bulk of fibre alone or some other factor is uncertain. Fibre creates a larger, softer stool that passes through the bowel more quickly and can also bind and inactivate potentially carcinogenic chemicals in the bowel. Recent studies have also shown that fibre is basically composed of a complex carbohydrate, glucan, which has been shown to have properties of stimulation of the immune (protective) system.

However, the results of various studies have been difficult to interpret. The exact role of fibre in the development of colorectal cancer is not clear. Again, a balanced diet remains an important general health recommendation.

Other dietary factors

Although the consumption of fruit and vegetables and some of their main micronutrients appears to have a role in cancer prevention, it does appear that it may be less important than previously thought. The evidence is still unclear, because some recent studies have documented a lack of association of these foods with the incidence of cancer. It is possible that increased intake of folic acid, a vitamin found in various fruits and vegetables, may play a role in cancer prevention. Other dietary ingredients for which cancer-protective properties have been claimed but are still inconclusive are antioxidants including betacarotene and retinol and trace elements selenium and zinc and also garlic. It is likely that a deficiency of some of these food ingredients might predispose people to carcinogenic changes but that additional cancer protection is not achieved by increasing the intake over and above what is in a healthy balanced diet. However, regardless of any cancer-preventing properties, a diet rich in fruit and vegetables is still recommended because of its beneficial effects in regard to heart disease, obesity and diabetes.

The different incidences of cancer of some tissues (e.g. breast and prostate) between Asians and Caucasians may also be related to diet. Traditionally Asians have a diet with a high content of legumes (peas, soybeans, etc.). Legumes contain considerable quantities of naturally occurring plant hormones, phyto-estrogens. Some studies suggest that this may be a factor in the relatively low incidence of breast diseases (including cancer) in Asian females and the relatively low incidence of prostate cancer in Asian males. This belief is supported by evidence that men and women of Asian races who are born and raised in Western countries, and Asian men and women who adopt Western diets, either in their own country or in a Western country, have a significantly increased risk of developing prostate cancer or breast cancer compared with those who keep to their traditional Asian diets. This risk in Asians who have changed to Western diets approaches the risk in Caucasians.

Another dietary factor of more recent interest is an antioxidant called lycopene.

Lycopene is in the red colouring ingredient of tomatoes. Experimental studies have shown that lycopene is protective against some cancers, especially breast and prostate cancers. This may help explain the lower incidence of both breast and prostate cancer in southern Europeans, who eat more tomato-containing foods than northern Europeans. Lycopene is better absorbed from cooked tomatoes, which is some comfort to those who love to eat pizzas and other foods containing tomato pastes or cover their foods with tomato sauces.

However, for most cancers there is little strong evidence that diet plays a part. There are so many variable factors among people of different population groups that it is always difficult to prove which particular factors are responsible for any difference in the incidence of cancer. As well as differences in diet there may be genetic differences, racial differences, environmental differences, or differences in social habits or customs such as smoking, differences in the incidence of parasites or infections, or even differences in occupational stress or psychological factors. The evidence of association between diet and cancer is strongest for cancer of the large bowel. Cancer of the oesophagus, stomach, pancreas and liver are all more common in heavy drinkers of alcohol, especially if they are smokers.

There have been theories that various vitamins may be protective against cancer. Although some of the claims of protection and cure with vitamins are exaggerated, there is some evidence that the antioxidant vitamins A and C may offer some protection. However, large doses of vitamin A can be harmful.

Members of the Seventh Day Adventist church have a lower than average incidence of most cancers, including cancers of the lung, oesophagus, stomach, pancreas, colon and rectum. However, as well as being vegetarians with a high-fibre diet and low meat and animal-fat consumption, these people are usually non-smokers and non-consumers of alcohol, which may well be more significant. A study of male members of the Seventh Day Adventist church is of interest. It was found that those church members whose diet included meat, eggs, cheese and milk had a greater incidence of cancer of the prostate than those who abstained from all animal products.

DOES RACE PLAY A PART?

Certainly some cancers are more prevalent in people of some races in their home countries than others. It now appears that this remarkable geographic variation in cancer risk largely reflects the effects of environmental differences. One such difference relates to personal habits such as smoking, betel-nut chewing, excessive alcohol consumption and recreational sun exposure. A further category reflecting environmental differences relates to the very common cancers involving the gastrointestinal tract and hormone-dependent female organs such as the breast, ovary, body of uterus and the prostate in men. Here the causes are less well defined and may reflect factors such as age at first pregnancy or dietary factors.

These conclusions are based on the changes seen when certain racial groups migrate to other countries and within a single generation there is a dramatic change in the incidence of various cancers. The best studied group have been the Japanese migrants, particularly to Hawaii and California. Here the incidence of gastric cancer falls rapidly, to be replaced by increasing incidence of colon and breast cancer. As well, the differences in risk for these cancers seen in Mormons and Seventh Day Adventists, as described above, relate to environmental differences.

Some examples of increased incidence are those of the higher frequency of gastric cancer in Japan, Korea, Scandinavia, Holland and Czechoslovakia, the high incidence of cancer of the oesophagus in certain African tribes (including the Bantu in South Africa) and also in Northern China. The high incidence of liver cancer (hepatoma) in the Shanghai area in China reflects a sequel of viral hepatitis, while in Africa it may be the result of a toxin taken in with food that causes liver cirrhosis. Breast cancer and large bowel cancer, of course, are much more common in people of European descent living in countries with a Western lifestyle and diet. People of Northern European descent with a fair complexion who indulge excessively in recreational sun exposure have a high incidence of skin cancers, including malignant melanoma.

DOES GEOGRAPHICAL LOCATION PLAY A PART?

The association of skin cancer and melanoma with fair-skinned people living in a sunny climate is obvious. The incidence is highest in fair-skinned people living in sunny climates in Australia and in the sunny southern parts of the USA. Australia not only has the world's highest incidence of skin cancer and melanoma, but the incidence varies from state to state according to proximity to the equator. For the more common forms of skin cancer (squamous- and basal-cell carcinoma) the incidence is directly related to areas of skin most exposed to the sun. Melanomas are most common on the back and chest in men and on the thighs and lower limbs in women. Clearly, for melanoma the cause is not only the amount of direct exposure of skin to sunlight. Some other factor associated with living in a sunny climate must play a part, one of which is skin damage caused by acute sunburn, especially if episodes of sunburn occurred in childhood.

Primary cancer of the liver (hepatoma) is common in South East Asia and East African countries, but this appears to reflect viral infection with hepatitis in Asia and in Africa, and aflatoxin produced by a fungal species contaminating foods. This also occurs in China. The cause of the high incidence of stomach cancer in Japan, Korea and Eastern European countries appears to be largely a dietary factor. This reflects food-handling practices and food-preservation techniques, as discussed earlier.

DOES ENVIRONMENT PLAY A PART?

Although for most cancers there is no apparent environmental factor, there are some important exceptions. The most obvious of these is the high incidence of skin cancers and melanoma among the white populations of Australia and the southern regions of the USA, caused by exposure to sunshine.

In Western societies, city dwellers living with air pollution have been found to have a slightly higher incidence of lung cancer than their country cousins. This factor, however, is not nearly as significant as the smoking habits of the people in these various environments.

The increased incidence of leukaemia in the survivors of the Hiroshima and Nagasaki atom-bomb explosions indicates the environmental effect of irradiation as a cause of this disease.

Burkitt's lymphoma, which predominantly affects children in tropical Africa and New Guinea, occurs in areas where mosquitoes are common and malaria is rife. The disease appears to reflect a sequel of Epstein-Barr viral infection in patients rendered immune deficient by chronic malaria.

Cancer of the thyroid is more frequent in communities where goitres are more common. Goitre (or thyroid-gland enlargement) is most common in areas where there is a deficiency of iodine in local food and water supplies. Such places are known as 'goitre belts' and are often in mountainous regions where iodine has been leached out of the soil over many years. These belts can be found in the Swiss Alps, the Rocky Mountains, the Andes, the Himalayas and the mountainous regions of New Guinea, Australia and New Zealand. The Great Lakes district in the USA is also a goitre belt. It is likely that the iodine has been washed out of the soil in the region into the Great Lakes and is lost through the rivers into the sea.

DOES OCCUPATION PLAY A PART?

Present-day industrial laws protect workers against most industrial dangers, including risk of exposure to cancer-causing agents. Before the effect of environment was understood, a number of cancers were linked with working conditions, but these have now been largely eliminated. For example, in the early days of X-rays, when doctors and technicians held the plates with bare hands, exposing them to repeated doses of radiation, there was a high incidence of skin cancer developing in the irradiated hands. Protection against such exposure to X-rays is now strictly monitored.

More recently (since the 1960s) awareness has grown of a highly malignant cancer of the lining of the lungs or abdominal organs called a mesothelioma in those exposed to asbestos. Even trivial exposure may sometimes lead to the development of such a tumour but often 20–40 years after the exposure. As well, asbestos workers in the past who were exposed to extremely high levels of asbestos were found, especially if they were smokers, to have an increased risk of developing lung cancer. Stringent improvements to working conditions have now been introduced to protect these workers.

Another, less obvious, risk is the increased incidence of cancer in the air passages behind and around the nose (the paranasal sinuses) in woodworkers, leather workers and metal workers, especially nickel workers. This is probably due to constantly breathing in small particles of these materials. There is also said to be an increased risk of cancer of the larynx in people who misuse their voices, such as old-time bookmakers who would shout a great deal in calling the odds, and in clergymen who spend long periods using a high-pitched chant. However, these risks would be very small compared to the risk of cigarette smokers developing the same sort of cancer.

DO HABITS AND LIFESTYLE PLAY A PART?

Certainly the most obvious carcinogen in present-day society is tobacco. Cigarette smoking outweighs all other known causes of serious cancer in men and women. The incidence of lung cancer is increased some tenfold to twentyfold in smokers compared with non-smokers. The risk is directly related to the amount of tobacco smoked in terms of both frequency and duration. In the past, the increased incidence of lung cancer was most obvious in men. In more recent years, with more women smoking, a dramatic increase is now occurring in women, as noted earlier.

Cancers of the mouth (oral cavity and tongue) and throat are also closely associated with the smoking habit. It is estimated that heavy smokers have about six times the risk of developing this form of cancer as non-smokers. The risk is increased many times over if the smokers are also heavy drinkers.

In the case of lung cancer the risk appears to be greater in cigarette smokers than in pipe or cigar smokers. However, for mouth cancers there is no apparent difference in risk between cigarettes, pipes or cigars. This is probably because cigarette smokers usually inhale smoke as well as collect some tobacco products in the mouth, whereas pipe and cigar smokers are less likely to inhale the smoke but do collect irritating tobacco carcinogens in the mouth.

Several other cancers have increased incidence in smokers, including cancers of the oesophagus, stomach, pancreas, kidney, bladder and even breast cancer.

Heavy alcohol drinkers also have an increased incidence of cancer of the mouth and throat, oesophagus, stomach, liver and pancreas. The risk is greater in those heavy drinkers who are also smokers.

Australians who spend most of their lives out of doors at work and play, on the beach and so on, are at greatest risk of developing basal and squamous skin cancers through cumulative exposure to the sun throughout life. However, melanomas appear to reflect sun exposure at a younger age, especially recreational exposure and individual episodes of sunburn. Paradoxically, outdoor workers have a lower incidence of melanoma, possibly reflecting the development of a protective tan that is not present in people who become intermittently sunburnt.

People in India or New Guinea who chew betel-nut or tobacco leaf have an increased incidence of cancer of the cheek lining.

The incidence of breast cancer is lowest in women who have their children at an early age. In communities where the custom is for women to marry early and have their first babies while they are still in their teens, the incidence of breast cancer is low, while in Westernised societies where first babies are commonly born to women over the age of 30 years, the incidence of breast cancer is higher. There may also be some protection against breast cancer in prolonged breastfeeding, as is common in most undeveloped countries, although the evidence for this is less clear. The reason for this lower risk of breast cancer is thought to be a reduction in the total duration of exposure to oestrogen.

The association of cancer with diet and eating habits has already been discussed.

There appears to be a direct relationship between the economic development of a country and the incidence of large-bowel cancer. In Australia and New Zealand it is the most common of all cancers other than skin cancer, and it is among the most common cancers in Europe and the USA. In many undeveloped countries it is rarely seen. A diet high in meat, animal fats and highly refined food as in Westernised, industrialised countries appears to produce cancer-inducing substances. The absence of fibre from the diet results in a relative constipation, which is thought to allow these carcinogens to stay in contact with the bowel wall for prolonged periods. In undeveloped countries the diet generally contains a great deal more roughage and fibre and less meat, fat and refined foods. This results in the passage of frequent bulky stools and a low incidence of large-bowel cancer. There are numerous examples to support this evidence. For example, Japanese who eat the traditional high-fibre diet in Japan have a low incidence of large-bowel cancer. However, in those who migrated to Hawaii or California and ate American food, the incidence of bowel cancer increased to virtually match that of Americans. Recent studies also suggest that starch-like substances called glucans may also have a protective action on the bowel wall. Glucans are found in such high-fibre foods as grains, fruit and vegetables, but there are few in fatty foods.

The naturally occurring plant hormones, phytoestrogens, which are present in large quantities in leguminous plants such as soybeans, are currently the subject of dietary studies. People who live in Asian countries where there is a high intake of these foods have a lower incidence of conditions that are common in Western societies, where the intake of phytoestrogens is low. These conditions include breast diseases such as cancer and premenstrual syndrome, as well as post-menopausal symptoms in women and prostate cancer in men.

Cultural and social customs may also have a relationship with the development of cancer. Cancer of the penis is extremely rare in Jewish men, who are circumcised at birth, but is seen more often in Muslim men who are circumcised at about ten years. The incidence is greatest in uncircumcised males.

Nuns have a low incidence of cancer of the cervix but an increased incidence of breast cancer. On the other hand, cancer of the cervix is most common in women who commence intercourse at an early age, and especially if they have had unprotected sex with multiple male partners. This risks a higher incidence of infection with the human papilloma virus (HPV). Women who have taken the contraceptive pill for some years appear to have a somewhat reduced chance of developing cancer of the ovary or uterus. However, prolonged use of contraceptive pills, especially the high-dose oestrogen pill, has been associated with a slightly higher risk of breast cancer. The small-dose oestrogen pill has not been shown to have any significant association with breast cancer.

DO PSYCHOLOGICAL FACTORS, STRESS OR EMOTION PLAY A PART?

Among the theories about cancer causation has been a suggestion that, as with emotional and some mental (psychosomatic) illnesses, cancer may result from an unnatural suppression of the 'fight or flight' response to anxiety or stress. It has been suggested that if a stressful situation persists over a long period and the person concerned feels that whatever action he or she takes will be wrong, a subconscious decision to escape through death by cancer may result. There is little evidence to support such a theory, although some retrospective studies have indicated that a significantly high proportion of cancer patients have experienced some form of severe stress in the period six months to two years before the onset of illness.

Most psychologists would not claim that psychological reactions are a direct cause of cancer, but some feel that they may play a part, possibly adding to the effects of the known chemical, genetic, environmental, viral or other causes. The association of possible psychological factors with cancer has indicated a need for additional psychological support by appropriate psychiatrists, clinical psychologists, social workers and/or other health workers. This association has also been put forward by a variety of 'fringe' medicine practitioners to justify their treatment practices.

CAN CANCER BE PREVENTED?

It is not possible to completely prevent people from developing a cancer at some stage in their life. However, it is obvious that the risk of many cancers can be considerably reduced by an appropriate lifestyle and screening for cancer or conditions that may lead to or be associated with cancer.

The most obvious measure to reduce the risk of serious cancer is to avoid smoking. By not smoking, the risk of developing many cancers, including lung cancer, mouth and throat cancer, cancers of the oesophagus, stomach and pancreas, is greatly reduced. Even breast cancer is more prevalent in long-term smokers. Passive smoking (spending frequent long periods in a smoky atmosphere) is also associated with increased cancer risk and should be avoided.

The risk of the common skin cancers (basal-cell carcinoma and squamous-cell carcinoma) can be greatly reduced by avoiding unnecessary direct exposure to sunshine or ultraviolet light. Nature's protection is pigment in the skin in coloured races, but for fair-skinned people protective clothing (long-sleeved shirts, wide-brimmed hats, etc.) and UV-blocking skin lotions offer considerable protection. The same measures may help to some extent in avoiding melanoma, although the direct effect of sunshine on exposed skin as a cause of melanoma is less clear. It seems that to help avoid melanoma intermittent episodes of sunburn should be avoided, especially in childhood.

Diets high in fibre, including cereals, fresh fruit and vegetables, and low in meat, animal fat, highly refined foods and chemically preserved foods offer some protection against the development of bowel, breast and prostate cancers. A physically active lifestyle is also helpful in this regard.

The addition of iodine to the diet (usually as iodised salt) in iodine-deficient goitre-belt areas may reduce the incidence of goitre and possibly of thyroid cancer. There is also some evidence that deficiency in the diet of the element selenium might predispose people to some cancers (e.g. breast, bowel or prostate cancers).

Encouragement of breastfeeding may possibly be helpful in reducing the incidence of breast cancer.

Industrial laws that protect workers from a number of known industrial cancer-causing agents play a significant role in cancer prevention. Many countries now have laws to protect people from the effects of passive smoking.

Treatment of any longstanding ulcers or chronically inflamed or irritated lesions may also be a protective measure against the development of cancer. This may affect a variety of lesions such as longstanding varicose ulcers; ulcers in the mouth possibly irritated by a jagged tooth or ill-fitting denture; gastric ulcers; ulcerative colitis of the colon or rectum; longstanding gallstones, kidney or bladder stones; chronically discharging bone infection (osteomyelitis) or prolonged irritation of a pigmented lesion on the skin.

Another preventive measure is to remove or otherwise properly treat other known pre-malignant conditions such as polyps, papillomas, hyperkeratotic skin lesions, leukoplakia in the mouth or moles that show any sign of irritation or change. Also removal of benign tumours that show any evidence of enlarging or which are known to have a risk of malignant change will reduce the danger of cancer developing. Such tumours might include adenomas in the parotid gland or thyroid gland; papillomas or adenomas in the breast; cysts in the ovary; papillomas or polyps in the colon, rectum or uterus; papillomas in the bladder; enlarging soft-tissue tumours of fat (lipomas), nerve tissue (neuromas) and muscle (myomas); tumours of blood or lymph vessels (haemangiomas or lymphangiomas); and occasionally tumours of cartilage (chondromas) or bone (osteomas).

People affected by familial polyps in the bowel (polyposis coli) will all eventually develop colon cancer if they live to middle age. This can be completely prevented by total removal of the colon and rectum in those people before cancer has developed. The recognition of inherited forms of cancer in certain families offers these individuals opportunities for screening and early detection. Similarly people should avail themselves of appropriate screening for breast, cervical, bowel and prostate cancer.

Until recently it has not been possible to immunise people against cancer, although immunisation against hepatitis B, which might predispose people to developing cancer in the liver, is possible and is recommended for people who live in or travel to countries where hepatitis B is prevalent. Recent studies in Australia by Professor Ian Frazer have shown that it may soon be possible to immunise all women against the human papilloma virus responsible for most cancers of the cervix. At present the immunisation is only given at no cost to girls and young women up to the age of 26.

2

presentation, tests and treatments for cancer

WHAT ARE THE SYMPTOMS OF CANCER?

Symptoms are complaints that cause a person to seek medical attention. Although it is true that a cancer may be present for some years before it causes symptoms, generally the earlier a patient seeks medical attention the greater the chance of curing the cancer.

Symptoms may result from two effects of a cancer: the local effects of the tumour itself or the effects of the cancer on the person as a whole.

Local symptoms

Usually local effects are noticed first. These might include one or more of the following: a lump; an ulcer that does not heal; pain; abnormal bleeding from the bowel, bladder, vagina or elsewhere; or interference of function of the organ or tissue involved. Such functional interference may be obstruction of the bowel in the case of bowel cancer, or a persistent cough or interference with breathing in the case of lung cancer. These symptoms of local trouble will depend on the position of the cancer, the organ or tissue in which it started, the type of cancer cells that have developed, the size of the tumour and the possible involvement of other organs or tissues near to the cancer.

General symptoms

The main general effects that may be noticed by a person with cancer are lassitude and loss of energy, loss of appetite, weight loss, the effects of blood loss or the effects of any spread of the cancer from where it started (primary site) to another organ or tissue (secondary or metastatic site). These are usually manifestations of advanced disease.

General effects may result not only from damage to or interference with function of the organ or tissue involved but also from the body's reaction to the presence of cancer.

Local and general features will be mentioned in more detail in Section 3, but some features are outlined below.

A lump, swelling or tumour of some kind is present in

virtually every cancer. The lump may be obvious if it is in the skin, the mouth or tongue, the breast, in lymph nodes under the skin, in fat or muscles (soft tissue), or can be felt on bone. On the other hand, not all lumps are malignant. In fact, most lumps are not malignant, but if a new lump is found anywhere in the body it is important to seek medical advice. The most common symptom of breast cancer, for example, is a lump in the breast. The lump is often found in the bath or shower, as it is more easily felt with soapy wet hands. (Women who carry out self-examination of the breasts while sitting or lying in the bath, using soapy wet fingers, sometimes detect a lump that may or may not be a cancer.)

An ulcer on the skin that does not heal quickly may be a cancer and should be examined by a doctor. Skin ulcers are usually obvious, but ulcers in the mouth or throat may be less obvious if they are painless. Any such ulcer should be examined by a doctor, especially if it has been present for more than a week or two with no evidence of healing. Most longstanding ulcers are not malignant. They may be caused by such conditions as varicose veins or poor arteries in the lower legs, or by jagged teeth, ill-fitting dentures or infections in the mouth. However, if there is any doubt, a doctor will arrange a biopsy. In a biopsy, a small piece of tissue is taken, usually from the edge of the ulcer, and examined by a pathologist under a microscope to determine its type and its cause.

Most cancers are painless early in the disease. Pain usually develops only after a cancer has become big enough to press on and damage surrounding tissues or nerves. In general, a small painless lump is more likely to be a cancer than a small painful lump, and it is not advisable to wait for pain to develop before seeking medical advice.

Bleeding may be a feature of many cancers of surface tissues. For some internal cancers (e.g. in the stomach, bowel, kidney, bladder, uterus or lung) bleeding is often the earliest feature. Any evidence of abnormal bleeding should be investigated. For example, with bleeding from the bowel, the blood might be bright red in colour (fresh blood) or it might be dark red or black, due to bleeding higher in the bowel or stomach and the blood undergoing partial digestion. Common symptoms in people with bowel cancer are those associated with anaemia, such as tiredness and pallor. This may reflect slow bleeding into the bowel and loss of iron from the body.

There may be blood in the urine, the vagina (especially between periods or after menopause), in the sputum (either from the mouth or throat or from the lung after coughing), from a mole on the skin or from a nipple. Although bleeding may be an indication of cancer, it does not always indicate cancer, as there are many other causes of bleeding. Bleeding or bruising at several sites or small haemorrhagic spots in the skin (petechial spots) may be an indication of a blood disorder, including those caused by leukaemias or lymphomas.

There may be interference with tissue or organ function. These symptoms vary a great deal depending on the site of a cancer. For example, a cancer in the mouth may make speaking or swallowing difficult. Cancer of the larynx will usually cause hoarseness or a change in voice. Cancer of the oesophagus is usually first noticed when there is difficulty with swallowing.

A cancer of the stomach may cause difficulty with eating, change in appetite or vomiting, and cancer of the bowel may cause a change in bowel habits (diarrhoea or constipation) or obstruct the bowel, causing abdominal pain, constipation and possibly vomiting.

Cancer of the prostate may interfere with passing urine. There may be difficulty in starting, more frequency in passing and possibly dribbling of urine after stopping urination. Occasionally there can be a complete blockage from passing urine, requiring urgent medical attention. Cancer of the bladder may cause similar symptoms, sometimes with blood in the urine.

Cancer of the lung may cause a persistent cough, local obstruction of air passages or local pneumonia, and cancers of the liver, bile ducts or pancreas may block the flow of bile from the liver, causing jaundice.

There are many other causes of these symptoms, but if any of these symptoms is noticed for the first time in someone who was otherwise well, and especially if the symptoms persist, they should be investigated by the patient's doctor.

Symptoms of secondary (metastatic) cancer

These symptoms will vary with the tissues or organs to which the cancer has spread. The most common site of spread is to nearby draining lymph nodes in the neck, armpits, groin or elsewhere. Enlargement of these nodes may sometimes be the first sign of the presence of a cancer nearby.

Spread of cancer to the liver from the bloodstream may cause jaundice or pain and swelling in the upper abdomen under the ribs on the right side. It may also lead to malnutrition, weight loss, or fluid collecting in, and possibly filling, the abdominal cavity (ascites).

Spread of cancer to the lungs may cause coughing, difficulty with breathing, fever, pneumonia or chest pain.

Spread of cancer to bones may cause pain or fracture in the bones. It may also cause anaemia due to destruction of the blood-forming bone-marrow tissues.

Spread of cancer to other soft tissues such as fat and muscles may cause swelling or lumps that may be felt under the skin.

Spread of cancer to the bowel or elsewhere in the abdominal cavity may cause bowel obstruction or swelling and fluid in the abdominal cavity.

Spread of cancer to the brain may cause severe headaches, vomiting, blurred vision, fits or unconsciousness. Some patients may even present as though they have had a stroke.

SIGNS OF CANCER

The abnormalities associated with cancer may have been noticed by the patient, in which case they are called symptoms. If they have not been noticed by the patient but have been found by the doctor, they are called signs. The doctor therefore looks for any of those features that may not have been noticed by the patient.

The doctor looks for local lumps or other abnormal swellings, ulcers, tender or painful areas, evidence of blood loss from bowel, urine, uterus, etc. and general effects on the patient such as weight loss and generally poor health. He or she also looks for evidence of spread to other organs or tissues, knowing the likely sites for spread from any particular type of cancer. Different cancers tend to spread to different organs or tissues.

The doctor knows the features of lumps that are most likely to be associated with cancer in general and with particular forms of cancer. For example, cancer lumps are usually harder than lumps from other causes. Cancer lumps usually are not cystic, i.e. fluid filled (although on occasions they may be), and they are usually not tender or painful unless quite advanced. As they enlarge, cancer lumps become adherent to nearby structures and therefore become less movable.

Cancer ulcers often have raised or heaped-up edges. They tend to grow into other tissues on which they lie, and there is usually surrounding swelling. They may bleed easily but usually not profusely. They may or may not be tender. Ulcers due to skin cancer are usually not tender, whereas malignant ulcers in the mouth and throat usually become quite tender in the later stages.

The doctor will also look for evidence of blood loss in the case of cancers in which bleeding is a likely feature. Blood in the faeces may be detected chemically even when it is not obvious to the naked eye (occult blood) and this may be an early feature of cancer of the stomach or bowel. In fact, occult blood loss in the stool is often used as a screening test for gastric or bowel cancer even if symptoms have not presented.

Blood in the urine may sometimes be found on microscopic examination when it is not obvious to the naked eye. This may be a feature of cancer of the kidney or bladder, although there are also other more common causes. The doctor will also carry out a general check for evidence of anaemia due to chronic blood loss. This special type of anaemia reflects a gradually worsening iron deficiency due to the continued low level of bleeding. In fact any adult in a Western society with iron deficiency, particularly a male, requires investigation of his or her bowel. The recommended frequency of investigations will depend on age, sex and any evidence of anaemia or unusual abdominal or bowel symptoms.

In looking for evidence of secondary spread of cancer, the doctor will first examine the draining lymph-node areas. For example, if a cancer in the head, mouth or throat region is suspected, the lymph nodes in the neck will be examined first. If breast cancer or cancer of the skin of the arm or chest wall is suspected, the lymph nodes in the armpits will be examined. If the cancer is thought to be in a lower limb or of the skin of the abdomen or lower back, scrotum, anus or vulva, the lymph nodes in the groin will be first examined.

Swollen abdominal lymph nodes may be the result of cancers of the stomach, pancreas, bowel, testes, uterus, ovaries or elsewhere in the abdominal cavity, but these usually can't be felt unless they are very large. They can be visualised by a special form of X-ray called a CT (computerised tomography) scan. (This was previously known as a CAT (computerised axial tomography) scan but is much more commonly known as a CT scan nowadays.) Sometimes lymphatic channels allow cancers to spread from the abdominal organs to the lymph nodes in the neck (usually the left side); these will be examined as they are easily felt if enlarged.

Cancers of the lung or the oesophagus often spread to lymph nodes in the chest, and although the swollen lymph nodes cannot be felt with the hands, evidence of their enlargement may sometimes be seen in a chest X-ray.

Lymph nodes may also be enlarged in malignant tumours known as lymphomas or leukaemias. If enlarged, these lymph nodes are usually somewhat rubbery and softer than nodes invaded by other cancers. They are also likely to be smoother in outline and are less likely to become fixed to other structures, and often lymph nodes on both sides of the neck or lymph nodes in other places may be involved. The spleen, which is an organ in the abdomen under the ribs on the left side, also behaves like a large lymph node, and although a normal spleen cannot be felt, it may become enlarged and palpable (easily felt) in these conditions.

The doctor will also look for evidence of lumps or swellings in other parts of the body, especially in the abdomen, the liver or other tissues or organs likely to be involved with any cancer.

Part of the examination of the alimentary (digestive) tract would be an examination of the mouth, tongue and throat as well as the anus. Most cancers of the rectum can be felt with a gloved finger in the rectum, and many other conditions, such as enlarged prostate, enlarged uterus or tumour in the pelvis, can be felt by this simple examination. Also, the colour and nature of the faeces and presence of blood in the faeces can often be detected from this examination.

WHICH TESTS HELP IN DETECTING CANCER?

A large range of tests is now available to help detect the various types of cancer. Some of the most useful have become available only during the past 20 years or so. They range from screening tests for detecting cancer in people at risk without any symptoms to organ imaging, in which X-rays, CT scans, ultrasounds, isotope scans, MRI and, more recently, PET scans may reveal the presence of internal cancers. There are also endoscopic tests in which flexible fibre-optic instruments allow doctors to look at, photograph and even biopsy lesions in the alimentary (digestive) tract, lung, airways, bladder or other body cavities. A number of blood and serum tests may reveal evidence of cancers releasing their own distinctive substances known as 'tumour markers'.

However, the most important investigation is a biopsy, in which a piece of tissue is examined under a microscope to determine whether or not a lesion contains malignant cells. The microscopic examination can very often also tell the exact type of malignant cells and the organ or tissue from which they originally developed. In the centre of all growing and mature cells is a cell nucleus that contains genes. Genes inherited from parents are responsible for the development of different body tissues and the functions and growth of each tissue. More recently, genetic material (DNA) from the biopsies can be tested for specific changes in the inherited genes (mutations). This can sometimes assist with diagnosis as well as with selecting the most appropriate treatments for individual patients.

Common screening tests
The cervical-smear or 'Pap' test

One of the first, and most useful, specific screening tests is the Papanicolaou or cervical-smear test for detecting early cancer at the entrance (neck or cervix) of the womb (uterus). Cancer of the cervix is the most common form of cancer of the uterus. Women over the age of 40 who have had pregnancies and/or several sexual partners are most at risk from this type of cancer. It is recommended that women have a cervical-smear test every second year. This has the advantage of being simple, painless, cheap and relatively reliable. In this test a swab or scraping is taken through the vagina from the cervix. Fluid from the swab or scraping is smeared over a glass slide and the slide is examined for cells by trained technicians. If malignant cells are found, cancer may be detected early and treated, with good results. Other abnormal cells may suggest changes that could go on to become cancer if not treated; simple treatment at that stage can prevent a cancer developing.

Breast screening

Cancer of the breast is the most common cancer in women in most Western societies. Although there is not one completely reliable screening test, a number of tests may be combined to detect early breast cancer. These include self-examination; examination for lumps in screening clinics by doctors or specially trained nurses; mammography (special breast X-rays); ultrasound studies; and biopsy using a fine needle to aspirate out fluid or cells from any suspicious lump. Any material aspirated is then examined under a microscope by a pathologist.

Occult blood tests

A number of chemical and other tests can be used to detect the presence of blood in the faeces where blood cannot be seen with the naked eye. The presence of blood in the faeces may indicate some abnormality in the stomach or bowel, and that abnormality may be a cancer or a pre-cancerous condition such as a polyp. This test is not always accurate, but it is sometimes used as a screening test to examine people who are most at risk of cancer and to detect those most in need of further tests. This is called a faecal occult blood (FOB) test.

Organ imaging tests
X-rays

Radiological studies or X-rays are a relatively old but useful method of medical examination for cancer. Techniques are constantly improving, and the doses of X-rays needed are becoming smaller and smaller. X-ray films are only able to detect spots or lesions that are different from the normal tissue in the region. This difference is seen as a relatively light or relatively dark shadow on a film. For example, X-rays pass easily through air in the lungs or gas in the large bowel, and this is shown as a dark shadow on a film. If a cancer is present in a chest X-ray, it might show as a relatively lighter or whiter part in the area normally showing as dark shadow from the air-filled lungs. On the other hand, X-rays are blocked by dense bone, which shows as a white area on film. If a cancer is present in bone, it may show as relatively dark or grey areas in the bone, which is otherwise white. Other tissues such as muscle and fat are intermediate between the dark shadow of air and the white shadow of bone in their penetration by X-rays. These tissues are of similar consistency and have similar penetration by X-rays as cancers, meaning it is not so easy to detect tumour shadows in soft tissues by this method; more sophisticated investigations may be required.

Barium, iodine compounds and some other materials (often called dyes) are not penetrated by X-rays, and these are often used in the body to outline cavities that are otherwise not easily seen on an X-ray film. After a patient swallows a barium mixture (called a barium meal) the dye will outline the shape of the stomach on an X-ray; if a cancer is present it may show as an abnormality in the shape or in the outline of the stomach. Similarly, a barium enema in the lower bowel may allow detection by X-rays of a cancer in the colon or rectum. These are less commonly done nowadays, however, given the availability of endoscopy.

An intravenous pyelogram (IVP) or excretory urogram involves the injection of iodine compounds into a vein. When these are passed through the kidneys into the urine and eventually flow into the bladder, they show the position, shape and size of the kidneys and the bladder in X-rays. Iodine compounds can also be injected into the bladder or the kidneys from below (through the urine pathway) and X-rays taken. Such X-ray studies of the kidneys are called retrograde pyelograms or retrograde urograms. This test can also be used for other body cavities such as the fluid-filled space around the spinal cord; an X-ray (called a myelogram) may show an abnormal outline if a tumour is present. However, this form of X-ray has been largely replaced by MRI (discussed later), which is more accurate and less invasive.

Some iodine compounds are also excreted in bile into the gall bladder and bile ducts. X-rays can then be used to outline the shape and contents of the gall bladder (cholecystogram) and bile ducts (cholangiogram), which again may show abnormalities if tumours or other defects, such as gallstones, are present. Again this form of examination is being superseded by sensitive ultrasound technology.

Screening

Whereas all X-rays were once recorded on film as still photographs, techniques now used allow the radiologist to study on a television screen the movement of a radio-opaque material (dye) such as barium or iodine in a body cavity. After a barium meal or barium enema the patient is taken into a dark screening room where the radiologist can change the position of the patient to allow the material to flow into various parts of the organ being examined and more accurately determine its size, shape, position and outline on the television screen. This way the radiologist can see if a lump in the bowel, for example, is a lump of faeces that can be moved through the bowel or if it is a tumour lump attached to the bowel wall.

Air, too, can be used to replace fluid in certain cavities and show up as shadows in X-rays. Air is sometimes used in the large bowel together with barium: the barium adheres to the wall of the bowel and the air fills the bowel cavity, allowing X-rays to show more precisely the shape of the wall of the bowel and any lumps projecting into the cavity. In the past, similar techniques were used in the brain, but these have been replaced by MRI.

In most cases, the X-ray density of a cancer is similar to the X-ray density of surrounding tissues, so X-ray films alone are unlikely to show evidence of a deep-seated cancer. For cancers that are not so deep-seated, however, such as breast cancer, X-rays (mammograms) may be used to detect any small differences in penetration of the tissues that may indicate the presence of a cancer.

Chest X-rays

Chest X-rays are most useful investigations for detecting abnormalities in the lungs, including cancers. These may show as white opacities in the dark, air-filled lungs, or the lungs or tissues between the lungs may be shown to be altered in size and shape. Lymph nodes in the chest are grouped around the midline between the lungs. If lymph nodes are enlarged, as with lymphomas, the centre area of white density in a chest X-ray may be widened.

Skeletal X-rays

Skeletal X-rays will show the outline and density of bones. Primary cancer of bone (i.e. cancer starting in the bone, called osteosarcoma) may sometimes be seen as an abnormal shape and abnormal density in one part of the bone, usually towards one or other end of a long bone. Secondary cancers in bone usually show as rounded, less dense areas in the bone or even as fractures. Some secondary cancers containing calcium may even show as rounded areas of increased density in the bone. However, X-rays are not infallible and will not always detect cancerous lesions in bone, especially if the lesions are small.

Mammograms

A mammogram is a special X-ray of the breast that may show the presence of cysts, fibrous tissue or a cancer in the less dense fatty tissue of the breast. Small amounts of X-rays only are needed, so this examination is safe if not used excessively and is especially useful as an aid to screening for breast cancer.

Angiography

Radio-opaque material (dye) may also be injected into arteries or veins, or even lymph vessels, for films to be taken or for immediate viewing on a television screen. The radiologist can then determine whether the vessels are in their normal position or whether they have been pushed aside by a lump that may, sometimes, be a cancer. Some cancers develop a distinctive blood supply that may also be detected by this technique.

Newer methods for angiography of arteries (arteriography) have allowed arteries in virtually every part of the body to be outlined by radiographic (X-ray) techniques. These methods may be helpful in detecting evidence of deep-seated cancers that are relatively inaccessible to most other methods of investigation. Again many of these investigations have been replaced by MRI imaging techniques, which are less invasive.

Isotope scans (or nuclear scintigraphy)

Isotope scans have some similarity to X-rays in that the shadows of a radioactive source are recorded on a film plate. In this case, the radioactive material is injected into a vein and distributed in the bloodstream. The radioactive dose used is very small and is made up of, or combined with, various agents depending on which organ or tissue is to be examined. Radioactive iodine, for example, is concentrated in the thyroid gland, and the amount of uptake, size, shape, position and consistency of tissue in the thyroid gland can be determined from such a test. Another such material is concentrated in bone, particularly in areas of the bone with cellular activity or growth. Thus a bone scan will not only outline the position, size and shape of the bone, but it will also show areas of abnormal cellular activity that may be due to cancer.

Similar scans are used to outline the size, shape and any abnormal activity of the liver and spleen. In these organs, cancer may show up as one or more areas of decreased activity. However, these approaches have been largely replaced by CT scans or by ultrasounds.

Similar radio-isotope scan tests are now available for a number of other organs or tissues, including the brain, lungs and lymph nodes.

Scanning is carried out with the patient lying on a special table. Apart from a needle prick to inject the material into a vein, it is a quite painless procedure.

CT scan

In the early 1970s British workers developed a technique in which small doses of X-rays were used to allow the build-up of a picture of tissues in cross-sections of the trunk, the head and neck or the limbs. By taking many cross-sectional pictures of the abdomen, for example, a three-dimensional reconstruction can be done by a sophisticated computer. The position, size and shape of all the organs, major blood vessels, bones and muscles in the abdomen can be seen, and the position, size and density of any abnormal tumour or swelling can be assessed with considerable accuracy. CT scanning requires highly specialised equipment and skilled personnel and is therefore relatively expensive. Although not an infallible investigation, it has proved to be of great value in investigating many cancers and tumours in otherwise inaccessible areas of the head, abdomen, chest or deep in the limbs.

CT scanning is carried out with the patient lying on a table and, like other types of X-rays, presents no discomfort to the patient except that of lying still for several minutes on a small foam mattress in a small confined space or chamber. Commonly the images are now recorded on a CD, which is much more convenient for both patients and doctors. The images can then be viewed on any personal computer or sent for second opinions by email, etc.

Ultrasound scans

X-rays, nuclear scans and CT scans all depend on the use of small doses of penetrating X-rays or gamma rays. Although these are safe if used with proper care, there are occasions when even these small doses are probably better avoided, particularly during pregnancy, as the developing foetus is highly sensitive to irradiation. It is also preferable not to expose the reproductive organs of those of childbearing age to X-rays.

In recent years, a technique using ultrasound waves has been developed to give a somewhat similar cross-sectional picture of body tissues and body organs to the CT scan. The principle depends on sound waves being reflected or bounced back in different degrees by body tissues of different density, somewhat like a sonar depth sounder. The ultrasound waves are quite harmless.

Ultrasound scans in general do not give as much information as CT scans but are more accurate in showing the position and type of some lesions. They may be used as an alternative to CT scans in some situations or in conjunction with CT scans in others.

Ultrasound examinations are quite painless and cause the patient no discomfort. They are safe to use in pregnancy.

MRI (magnetic resonance imaging) scans

MRI can also show tissue on a cross-sectional film picture. Although an MRI is similar in appearance to a CT scan, it is based on quite different principles of physics. The scanning machine creates a strong magnetic field. Minute particles (atomic nuclei) in various tissues attempt to align themselves in the magnetic field and rotate or spin. This can emit energy detected by the scanner, creating images of organs and abnormal tissues. In some body tissues such as those in bone, muscle and in the brain and cranial cavity (skull box) an MRI scan may show more detail and information than a CT scan. Sometimes both studies are used and together they may complement each other in giving slightly different information about the size, shape and other characteristics of a tumour and the extent of its spread in surrounding tissues. As with CT scanning, the patient feels no pain but is required to lie still on a firm table and in a confined space for several minutes. Some patients find this claustrophobic. MRI scans are of particular value in investigating tumours of the brain and spinal cord as well as musculoskeletal disease. Because of the strong magnetic fields involved, MRIs should not be used on people with a cardiac pacemaker.

PET (positron emission tomography) scans

The PET scan is the most recent of all non-invasive studies (studies that do not require an instrument to be put inside the body, or a piece of tissue removed or a surgical operation). This remarkable but very costly scan is available in an increasing number of specialised centres. PET scanning is still the subject of ongoing research to determine exactly how it can help in the diagnosis and treatment of cancers and other serious medical conditions.

PET scans are quite different from X-rays, CT or MRI studies. X-rays are used to produce films that show as black and white shadows with shades of grey. These are inexpensive and readily available but do not give nearly as much information as CT or MRI films. Both CT and MRI scans give more three-dimensional information about the position, size, shape and consistency of tumours or lumps deep to the surface and their position in relation to other tissues such as arteries, nerves, muscles, bone and important organs. They are also produced in black and white pictures with shades of grey. They are based on laws of physics using penetration of X-rays and other rays under different conditions, including a change in magnetic fields in the case of MRI.

Although PET scans produce three-dimensional pictures that may be in black and white or in colour, they are based on different chemical activity in different types of tissues and different cells. The basic principle is that cancer cells use more glucose than normal cells: PET scans show areas of different glucose activity in body tissues and are often able to show the activity of the cancer, such as its rate of growth and any changes made by treatment given. They are better able to show whether some cancers have spread to other places. This is very important in determining the operability of certain cancers. They may also indicate whether a cancer has responded to treatment or whether it might be starting to come back again (relapse) after treatment.

PET scanning is a very safe procedure, but it is expensive. Its role is increasing but still limited to certain cancer types and situations.

Endoscopic examinations

Most people are familiar with a dentist using a mirror to examine the back of the teeth and a doctor using a head mirror to reflect light waves into the mouth to examine the throat, larynx or back of the nose. In recent years, the principle of using mirrors and lenses with a light source to examine the inside of body cavities has been refined to degrees of precision not considered feasible a decade or two ago. Previously, non-operative examination of the inside of body cavities was limited to examination of the larynx, trachea and air passages (bronchi), oesophagus, stomach, rectum and lower large bowel, bladder and vagina through rigid or semi-rigid tubes. These are still useful methods of examination, as they allow ready examination of these organs. They are reasonably simple to use, reasonably cheap to buy and are readily available either in doctors' surgeries or in hospitals.

Sigmoidoscopy

Although largely replaced by a more flexible colonoscope, a sigmoidoscope can still perform a valuable examination for large-bowel cancer. About 50% of all large-bowel cancers are within reach of a rigid sigmoidoscope. Sigmoidoscopy can be done in a doctor's surgery without anaesthesia, and a biopsy of any suspicious tissue can be taken at the time of examination. Some precautions are first taken to empty the bowel. The patient usually lies on one side and the sigmoidoscope is passed through the anus. Air is blown into the bowel to inflate it and so open up the lumen or bowel cavity. This air and the passage of the instrument is uncomfortable, but not unbearably so. Recently flexible sigmoidoscopes have been developed, which has simplified this procedure.

Proctoscopy

Examination of the anus and lower rectum can be carried out quite simply in a doctor's surgery with a small metal tube-like instrument called a proctoscope or anal speculum. Although it does not penetrate far into the rectum, it can be useful for detecting or treating lesions in or near the anus, such as haemorrhoids or cancer of the anus, which is rather rare.

Vaginal speculum

A vaginal speculum is a metal instrument that allows a doctor to examine the walls of the vagina or cervix in the surgery without significant discomfort to the patient. This speculum is used when Pap smears are done.

Laryngoscopy and bronchoscopy

The larynx may be examined indirectly with a mirror in the doctor's surgery, but a more direct examination of the sensitive larynx or main air passages is usually carried out with a flexible fibre-optic laryngoscope or bronchoscope in hospital with sedation and local anaesthetic sprays.

Oesophagoscopy

Examinations of the oesophagus in the past have usually been carried out in hospital under general anaesthesia using rigid instruments. Today flexible scopes are available, and with simple sedation and sprayed local anaesthetics the procedure is not painful or distressing.

Cystoscopy

The bladder may be examined with a rigid cystoscope, usually in hospital under general anaesthesia.

Flexible scopes

Advances have been made with flexible instruments using fibre-optic technology. These instruments have virtually replaced the older rigid scopes. The newer scopes allow digital photos or videos to be taken as well as biopsies.

Gastroscopy (endoscopy)

Expert gastroenterologists can pass modern gastroscopes through the patient's mouth into the stomach without general anaesthesia, provided the patient is suitably sedated. They are passed with little discomfort. Gastroscopes (endoscopes) allow examination not only of the oesophagus and stomach but also of the first part of the small bowel (duodenum). Through the duodenum they also allow examination of the opening of the bile duct from the liver and gall bladder, and the pancreatic duct from the pancreas. Radio-opaque material can be injected into these ducts, allowing X-rays to be taken for more detailed examination.

Colonoscopy

The colonoscope is a flexible instrument that can be passed through the anus and around the whole length of the large bowel to allow its examination. The instrument can be used to detect and remove pre-malignant polyps or to take biopsies. Special preparation is required to empty the bowel before the colonoscope is used. This instrument may be passed without undue discomfort if the patient is well sedated, although some patients may prefer general anaesthesia.

Peritonoscopy (laparoscopy) and thoracoscopy

The body cavities – the peritoneal cavity of the abdomen and the thoracic or pleural cavities of the chest – may also be examined by passing instruments called a peritoneoscope or thoracoscope through a small incision ('key hole') into the cavity. This is carried out under general anaesthesia in the operating theatre. In some situations biopsies may be taken. Special equipment is now available to carry out some surgical operations using similar scopes, with surgical instruments passed through a second small opening in the abdominal or chest wall. Certain cancer operations in the chest or abdomen can be carried out in this way.

Culdoscopy

Culdoscopy is an examination of the pelvis. The instrument is passed into the pelvic cavity through a small incision made in the top of the back wall of the vagina.

Bronchoscopy

With a flexible instrument the trachea and larger airways (bronchi) can be visualised and biopsies or cell brushings can be obtained. This examination is commonly used when lung cancer is suspected.

Blood and serum tests

Blood tests may show either direct or indirect evidence of cancer.

Haemoglobin and red-cell count

Most cancers eventually cause some degree of anaemia, and

haemoglobin and red-blood-cell counts will show evidence of this. Some cancers might be quite advanced, however, before evidence of anaemia is present. If the anaemia tests show that it is being caused by iron deficiency, especially in an adult male or post-menopausal woman, a bowel cancer is often suspected as the likely underlying factor. This is then investigated with a colonoscopy. Iron-deficiency anaemia is diagnosed by finding red cells that are small and contain low amounts of haemoglobin and a low Ferritin level (a measure of iron stores) in the serum.

White-cell count

The white-cell count may also be affected in some types of cancer. More significantly, examination of the number and type of white cells may show the first evidence of a leukaemia or lymphoma.

Serum biochemistry

Some types of cancer are likely to change biochemical components in the blood. For example, cancer of the prostate gland may result in an elevation of the enzyme called serum alkaline phosphatase; advanced breast cancer may cause elevation of serum calcium; and a particular type of large-bowel cancer may cause loss of potassium from the bowel, causing a fall in serum potassium. Cancers in the liver may cause a degree of liver failure, which may also be detected by changes in serum biochemistry.

Tumour markers

Cancer researchers have been looking for some years to find some specific biochemical product in the blood as a result of a cancer or the body's reactions to a cancer. Some research involved the study of immune reactions in the body to the presence of cancer. The most widely used of these tests are the serum carcino-embryonic antigen (CEA), the alpha-feto-protein, beta chorionic gonadotropin (b-hCG) and prostate specific antigen (PSA) tests.

A CEA test looks for the presence of CEA in blood. CEA is released from certain cancers, especially those of the large bowel and other forms of adenocarcinoma (glandular cancers). A high level or titre of this material may suggest the presence of bowel cancer, and a return to a low level after treatment may indicate that most or all of the cancer has been eradicated.

The alpha-feto-protein test is similar and may indicate the presence of a primary liver cancer called hepatoma or a testicular cancer. Similarly the b-hCG test is of value in testicular cancer diagnosis and monitoring successful or unsuccessful response and results of treatment.

A PSA test is a blood test that may indicate abnormality of the prostate gland in men. Sometimes this abnormality may be cancer of the prostate, especially if the level of PSA is high. A return to low levels after treatment may indicate that the cancer has been eradicated and the patient possibly cured. There is some controversy at present regarding the use of this test to screen for prostate cancer (as discussed in Section 3 under 'Cancer of the prostate').

Tumour-marker tests are not totally reliable, but a great deal of work is being carried out in this field. Other blood-test markers are sometimes used in breast, ovarian, biliary and pancreatic cancers.

Biopsy

The most reliable test for cancer is the tissue biopsy, in which a piece of tissue is taken from a suspected cancer and examined under a microscope. Provided a proper sample of tissue is taken, examination of the cells in the biopsy specimen will usually allow a pathologist to determine not only whether a cancer is present but also the type of cancer, the tissue of origin of the cancer and even the degree of malignancy. Sometimes the biopsy may also give a good indication of the likelihood of a cure.

Incision and excision biopsies

Biopsies are usually taken by a surgeon at operation. The surgeon will take a small representative sample of a suspected cancer (incision biopsy) or, if the tumour is small, the whole tumour will be removed for examination (excision biopsy).

A number of techniques have been developed to assist a diagnosis by biopsy.

Needle-aspiration or punch-out biopsy

For some tumours (e.g. some lumps in the breast) it is possible to insert a special needle into the lump and aspirate or suck out sufficient cells or tissue for biopsy examination (needle-aspiration biopsy). There is also a special needle called 'Trucut' with a mechanism that allows a small core of tissue to be punched out (punch-out biopsy). This might be done under local anaesthesia without admission to hospital. These biopsies may be done with visualisation of the tumour using either ultrasound or CT scanning. Provided a correct specimen is taken and an expert pathologist is available to examine it, a diagnosis can be made rapidly with little disturbance to the patient.

Needle-aspiration or punch-out biopsy may now be used for a number of different types of tumour in a variety of other tissues such as the prostate gland, the liver and the thyroid gland, and deep-seated tumours in the limbs or chest.

Aspiration cytology

Aspiration cytology is similar to aspiration biopsy, except that it also applies to examination for cells in cysts or other fluid. A cyst in the breast or elsewhere may be aspirated and, by special preparation, the contents can be examined for the presence of malignant cells. If malignant cells are found, a diagnosis of cancer can be made. If, however, no malignant cells are found, there may still be some chance that cancer is present. It is possible that cancer cells could be in the cyst but not in the sample of fluid taken.

Bone-marrow biopsy

A similar aspiration technique is used in bone-marrow biopsy to obtain specimens of bone marrow for determining the presence and type of suspected leukaemia and other diseases involving the bone marrow, including secondary cancer or lymphoma.

Frozen-section biopsy

Frozen-section biopsy is a technique used to prepare biopsy specimens for examination quickly. Usually, the preparation and staining of a biopsy specimen for microscopic examination takes three or four days, sometimes even longer. The tissue is prepared, embedded in a wax block and stained in different ways to reveal special features of the cells. For some tumours it may be important for the surgeon to know the diagnosis immediately, so that any necessary cancer operation can be completed without delay. By using the technique of frozen section, in which the biopsy specimen is prepared by immediately being frozen solid and then stained, the pathologist may be able to give the surgeon an accurate diagnosis within a few minutes. If the patient is anaesthetised and prepared for operation, the surgeon may be able to completely remove the cancer at the same operation. Frozen-section techniques are now highly accurate for most cancers if used by skilled pathologists, but in some cases it may not be possible to make an accurate diagnosis until special pathology sections have been prepared in the usual way, by embedding the tissue specimen in wax. Now, with advances in biology, many other tests are done on the biopsy using special antibodies or DNA (gene) expression or mutation tests. These help further in designing the best treatment for the patient.

CAN CANCER BE CURED?

Although cancer is a frightening word, in modern developed societies 50–60% of the more serious cancers are cured. That figure does not include the small skin cancers that are so common in older age in fair-skinned people who live in sunny climates, almost all of which are cured. The curability of a cancer depends on the type of cancer and the tissue from which it has grown, the position of the cancer in the body, the degree of abnormality of the individual cancer cells, the size of the cancer, the structures into which it may have grown and the presence and site of any secondary spread of the cancer. The age and general health of the patient may also be of significance. The patient's natural defence reactions are probably significant too. However, this is not clearly understood and not yet able to be appropriately measured.

Many of the most significant factors will depend on the stage at which the cancer is detected and treated. A small cancer detected early, before it has spread or involved other tissues, may be eminently curable, whereas the same cancer, enlarged and spread to other sites, may be quite incurable. However, the inherent aggressiveness of a particular cancer is critical in terms of outcome.

The best chance of curing cancer lies in the hands of the therapist or team of therapists who make the first attempt. That is, a cancer that has recurred after a failed attempt at treatment is more difficult to cure than it would have been at the first attempt. The quality of treatment given to the patient, especially in the initial treatment, is therefore a most important factor in determining whether or not a cure is likely to result. Commonly, doctors work in so-called multidisciplinary teams. These comprise surgeons or surgical oncologists, radiotherapists and medical oncologists.

In Western societies some of the most common cancers are basal-cell and squamous-cell cancers of the skin. Not only do these cancers grow relatively slowly and rarely spread, they are obvious to the patient and doctor when they are quite small and if properly treated at that stage are eminently curable. However, even disregarding basal-cell and squamous-cell carcinomas, more than half of all patients with more serious cancers can now be cured. Even the more aggressive and dangerous pigmented skin cancer, the melanoma, is usually quite curable in its early stages. With people becoming more aware of the danger of any change in a pigmented mole, or other dark spot on the skin, most melanomas are now detected and cured before they have spread.

The cancers that are least likely to be cured are often those that develop in deep body tissues and are not usually obvious until they have reached a stage when they have spread to lymph nodes or other tissues. These include cancer of the oesophagus, stomach, pancreas and lung. Hence there is a search on for methods of early detection for these cancers. Other cancers with poor prognosis include those in organs that cannot easily be dispensed with, such as the liver or brain. Until recently, cancers that developed in cells scattered widely throughout the body tissues, such as the lymphomas and leukaemias, were considered incurable, but with modern treatment methods increasing numbers of patients with these malignancies are also being cured.

The common cancers of the breast, prostate and bowel, and cancers of the uterus, are somewhat intermediate in their prognosis. It is most important that these cancers are detected early, as the outlook is much better if treatment starts when they are small. For this reason, cancer-screening clinics have been established to detect potentially curable cancers before they reach an incurable stage.

WHAT TREATMENTS ARE AVAILABLE?

Cancer prevention

As for all health problems (growing old excepted) prevention is better than cure. There are seven mainstays of cancer prevention. These are:

(1) Avoid both smoking and an excessively smoky atmosphere.

(2) Protect skin against excessive sunshine.

(3) Follow a simple diet low in animal fat and high in fresh fruit and vegetables, grains and fibre (as outlined below).

(4) Perform regular self-examinations to watch for any pre-cancerous lesions such as a breast lump or an abnormally pigmented or non-healing skin lesion.

(5) Attend screening tests to detect and treat any prevalent cancer in the community, such as breast, prostate and bowel cancer, melanoma and cancer of the cervix.

(6) See your doctor if you notice something different appearing and/or developing.

(7) Encourage and support safe industrial practices, and limit exposure to atmospheric pollution, carcinogens or irradiation.

An eighth important part of cancer prevention is the soon to be widely available immunisation against the human papilloma virus, which is making cancer of the uterine cervix a largely preventable disease.

Dietary advice

An important dietary factor that has captured a great deal of interest has been the apparent protective value of diets with a high content of plant hormones, phytoestrogens, in the daily diet, as previously discussed.

It is also likely that other plant products, possibly some with antioxidant properties and certain ingredients of some green vegetables, may have other anti-cancer biological actions in human and animal tissues. Some foods presently under study include cabbage, Brussels sprouts and broccoli, nuts, grains, red wine and lycopene (the red colouring antioxidant in tomatoes and other red fruits).

Another major piece of dietary advice is to avoid obesity. Overweight people are more prone to many health problems, including cancer.

Therefore, a good simple diet and regular exercise program is good advice for all, but it is especially advisable for infants and children to follow from early in life. It seems likely, however, that such dietary and exercise practices are cancer preventive but not curative.

The three mainstays of treatment of established cancer are surgery, radiotherapy and chemotherapy, including endocrine and biologic therapies.

Surgery

Surgery is the oldest and still the most important form of cancer treatment. The surgeon's objective is to excise the cancer in its entirety, together with all adjacent tissues into which cancer cells may have become attached or spread. For some types of cancer, especially for early skin cancers and small cancers in the mouth, surgery offers a relatively simple, straightforward, quick and effective treatment method. For cancers that may have spread to draining lymph nodes, the surgeon removes not only the primary cancer but all draining lymph nodes most likely to be involved. The primary cancer and lymph nodes are sometimes removed in one block of tissue. If a great deal of tissue has to be removed, the surgeon may need to do some form of plastic or reconstructive procedure to leave as little defect or deformity as possible.

More recently the concept of sentinel-lymph-node biopsy has come under investigation. Here, especially for breast cancer or melanoma, the first draining lymph node or nodes are identified by injection into nearby skin of either a dye or a radiotracer. These isolated, often single, nodes are then surgically excised and sent to pathology. In some patients this might indicate the need for a less radical operation than might otherwise have been considered necessary.

For breast cancer that is confined to the breast, with possible early involvement of lymph nodes in the axilla (armpit), a total removal of the involved breast and lymph nodes from the armpit as one block of tissue (radical mastectomy) was originally performed. Over the last 20–30 years an alternative for certain types of breast cancer has been local removal of the cancer, leaving the breast relatively intact. However, radiotherapy to the breast is then usually required.

For deep-seated cancers the whole or part of the involved organ is usually excised together with nearby draining lymph nodes. This is standard treatment for cancer of the stomach, colon, rectum, uterus, oesophagus, lung, kidney and sometimes pancreas.

Sarcomas in limbs tend to recur unless widely excised, and often the best chance of cure by surgery, especially for big sarcomas, is by the amputation of an affected limb. However, newer combined treatment techniques (see below) have reduced the need for amputation in many cases.

Radiotherapy

Radiotherapy is the second-oldest effective form of treatment for cancer in developed societies. It was introduced in the early years of the twentieth century with, at that time, very primitive equipment producing X-rays. Treatment today depends on the sensitivity of dividing cells to electron beams generated by linear accelerators. Treatment, equipment and techniques are constantly being improved, with better results in eradicating cancer cells and causing less damage to surrounding tissues and cells. The equipment is controlled by special computers planning the treatment targets (fields), with the aid of CT scans.

Radiotherapy may, in some cases, avert a surgical operation, but in many cases treatment over three, four or five weeks is required. It is often used before or after surgery in 'multimodality therapy'. It also has the disadvantage of causing some damage to normal tissues and cells surrounding the cancer in the area treated (the irradiation field). The objective of the radiotherapist is to position the patient and the radiation fields in such a way as to include all the cancer in the radiation field, with minimal exposure of normal tissue, thus achieving greatest destruction of cancer cells with as little damage to normal tissues and cells as possible.

Radiotherapy is effective treatment for many skin, mouth and throat cancers and for some deep-seated cancers that cannot be totally removed by surgery. It is also used as a palliative treatment to reduce the size of some cancers that cannot be cured by other means.

The dose of radiotherapy used is critical and must be determined by experts. Too little will not destroy cancer cells, but too much will destroy normal tissues and may result in painful ulcers that may not heal and other long-term local problems. The dose is also cumulative: once radiotherapy has been given to a part of the body in a treatment dose, it cannot be given again to the same site without risk of serious tissue damage.

Radiotherapy is quite painless, although it may leave some skin changes resembling sunburn and the patient may feel listless and tired after treatment. Although the red flush of skin change settles after a few weeks, some minor skin changes with small, dilated blood vessels are often a permanent feature of an area that has been irradiated.

For advanced cancers radiotherapy may be integrated with chemotherapy and/or surgery to achieve greater and more effective eradication of cancer cells (as discussed in the next section).

Chemotherapy

Doctors, scientists and others have been searching over the centuries for chemical substances that might cure cancer. The effect of some naturally occurring hormones in depressing the growth of certain cancers was first noticed early last century, but it was only in 1945, when it was observed that mustard gas destroyed dividing cells, that nitrogen mustard was discovered as a drug that could be used clinically against cancer cells. Many effective anti-cancer drugs have been developed since that time. These drugs have their greatest effect on dividing cells: as cancer cells divide much more frequently than normal body cells, they are more likely to be affected than the normal cells. The present anti-cancer drugs are grouped or classified according to the manner in which they affect dividing cells. They act on different components within the cancer cells, including DNA, the micro-tubules, chromosomes and others.

The more commonly used drugs fall into specific classes. Some of the most important of these are the so-called alkylating agents. These drugs can be given orally or intravenously, and they form a clinical bond with the DNA strands in the chromosomes. When the cell goes to replicate its DNA in the process of dividing, the interaction with the drug causes the strands to break and kill the cells. The drugs included are cyclophosphamide, melphalan, busulphan and chlorambucil. Their major side effects can include hair loss and a fall in the white-cell count. Similarly the drug cisplatinum, which is derived from the metal platinum, also binds to DNA in cancer cells, causing DNA breaks and cell death. It was first discovered in the 1970s and has proven to be curative in testicular cancer. It is also used in treating a wide range of other cancers (e.g. breast, lung and head and neck), often in combination with other drugs.

Another major class are the so-called antimetabolites. The commonly used drugs in this class are fluorouracil, methotrexate, gemcitabine and cytosine arabinoside. These drugs are very similar in structure to normally occurring biochemical intermediates that lead to the synthesis of DNA. The antimetabolites inhibit many of these steps, preventing the cell from replicating its DNA and therefore from being able to divide.

There are other classes of drugs. The so-called microtubule agents prevent the proper assembly of chromosomes at cell division. The chromosomes are supported by a scaffolding that is made up of a series of small elements rather like doughnuts. The drugs that inhibit this process are often derived from natural products, such as the drugs vincristine, vinblastine and vinorelbine, as well as the taxane class of drugs. Another major group are the anthracyclines. These are large, highly coloured molecules that also bind to DNA. They are extensively used in breast cancer and lymphoma treatment.

In treating cancers, the specialist cancer clinician (oncologist) selects drugs that are known to be effective against the type of cancer being treated with the least possible damage to normal body cells. In general, appropriate combinations of drugs are more effective than large doses of one drug only, and much research is being done to discover the most effective and safe combinations, doses and timing schedules of drugs against different types of cancer. For some cancer types, including lymphoma, testis cancer, leukaemia and children's cancer, chemotherapy of various types given alone may be curative.

Palliative chemotherapy

A common use of anti-cancer drugs is in treating advanced or metastatic cancers that cannot be treated effectively by surgery or by radiotherapy. Although some cancers can be cured by drugs, in general this form of treatment is palliative. (Palliation means that the cancer may be reduced in size and the patient given relief of symptoms for some time, but almost invariably the cancer will recur sooner or later and eventually death from the cancer, after a period of months or some years, is likely.)

Palliative chemotherapy, by reducing the cancer, will usually prolong life and make the patient more comfortable. Sometimes, however, because of the inconvenience and problems associated with treatment and the possible distress of side effects (see below) there is doubt as to whether palliative chemotherapy is worthwhile. In each case the doctors should discuss the likely benefits and possible problems with the patient and his or her family before a final decision is made about the treatment. Although it is the doctor's responsibility to give informed advice, the final decision as to whether or not to have palliative chemotherapy should be made by the patient. If doubt exists in the patient's mind about such treatment, a trial course may be appropriate; that is, treatment begun with the proviso that if the patient finds it too distressing, it can be modified or stopped at any time.

Adjuvant chemotherapy

More recently anti-cancer drugs have been used to destroy any cancer cells that may remain in the body after all obvious cancer cells have been removed, usually by surgery. Anti-cancer drugs are given after surgery in cancers where it is known there is a significant risk that scattered cancer cells may be present, even though they cannot be detected.

At present the most common use of adjuvant chemotherapy

is in treating women who have had a breast cancer treated by surgery (mastectomy) and in patients with colon or rectal cancers. A rarer but important use is after surgery for osteosarcoma (bone cancer) and cancers in young children.

Regional chemotherapy

Although surgery is limited to treating cancers localised to a particular region that can be excised, and radiotherapy is limited to treating cancer cells in a limited radiation field, chemotherapy is generally given systemically, that is, to the body as a whole. Anti-cancer drugs are sometimes given by mouth or more commonly by injection into a vein. The drug is absorbed into the bloodstream and distributed by the blood to all parts of the body.

When cancers are limited to one particular region of the body and that region is supplied with blood by one particular artery, it is sometimes possible to concentrate the anti-cancer drugs on the cancer by injecting or infusing the drugs directly into that artery. This is called regional or intra-arterial chemotherapy.

Sequential-combined-modality treatment

For relatively small and relatively uncomplicated localised cancers that can be effectively treated by surgery or radiotherapy, these forms of treatment are best used in a straightforward and usually simple fashion.

For some cancers, however, surgery alone or radiotherapy alone may not be able to provide a cure, or a surgical operation required to eradicate the cancer may be so mutilating as to be unacceptable to the patient. In these circumstances better results can sometimes be achieved by combining surgery and/or radiotherapy and/or chemotherapy in sequence.

Present-day treatment of some breast and bowel cancers is an example of a widely accepted use of combined treatment. For women with moderately advanced breast cancer the breast and axillary (armpit) lymph nodes are usually removed surgically. Nearby lymph nodes that have not been removed at operation may be treated by radiotherapy, but adjuvant chemotherapy is given (by intravenous injections) to control any cancer that may have escaped in the circulation and caused growths in other organs or tissues. Hormone therapy may also be used, either following chemotherapy or as an alternative.

An exciting new advance in the treatment of breast cancer after surgery is the use of an antibody directed against a high-intensity growth-signal receptor (HER2) on the surface of the breast cancer cells in about 20% of patients. This antibody is called Herceptin but is extremely expensive at this time.

Induction (neoadjuvant) chemotherapy

In treating some cancers that appear to remain localised to the site of origin but are unlikely to be cured by surgery or radiotherapy alone, another form of combined treatment is sometimes successful. In these situations the chemotherapy is best given first to reduce the size and extent of the cancer and to reduce its ability to grow and spread. It may then be possible to totally remove the reduced cancer by either surgery or radiotherapy. If the prospects of cure by either surgery or radiotherapy are still not good, it is often possible to use both radiotherapy and surgery after the chemotherapy. Work in this form of combined treatment is showing encouraging results, especially with some cancers in the head and neck (including the mouth and throat), some cancers in the stomach, some breast cancers and some cancers and sarcomas in limbs. In these situations it may be possible to give the chemotherapy more effectively by using the intra-arterial-infusion technique of regional chemotherapy (discussed above). Certain patients with rectal cancers are treated with combined chemo/radiotherapy prior to surgery. This may reduce the need for a colostomy and reduce the chance of local cancer recurrence.

Side effects of chemotherapy

The risk of using cytotoxic anti-cancer drugs is that as well as killing cancer cells they also cause damage to normal body cells. As with radiotherapy, the doses given and methods of administration must be arranged by experts familiar with their use so that maximum damage to cancer cells with minimum damage to normal cells and body tissues will result. Cells that are dividing are the most susceptible to these agents. Cancer cells, which are constantly dividing, are therefore more susceptible than normal cells. However, a number of cells in normal tissues divide frequently to repair and replace tissues and cells that are constantly being worn out or lost. These include blood-forming cells (in the bone marrow), surface skin and hair cells, cells lining the mouth, throat, stomach and bowel, and cells lining the air passages. The most serious side effect of most anti-cancer agents is a fall in the white cells or platelets in the blood: this may lead to a reduced resistance to infection or to bleeding. Regular blood counts are taken to determine whether the doses of drugs may need to be adjusted. In certain situations cytokines produced by gene-engineered biotech processes can prevent or reverse these falls in the white-cell count. Other possible side effects are mouth and throat ulcers, nausea and vomiting, hair loss or bleeding from the bowel. While some of these side effects are common, they are all reversible after the drugs have been stopped. There are now very effective medications to prevent nausea or vomiting after chemotherapy.

A small number of anti-cancer drugs may affect the function of the heart or lungs or nerves, but these effects are not often seen as they are unlikely to occur with normal doses of the drugs. However, doctors still watch closely, and at any sign of these problems these drugs are stopped. Certain tests of cardiac function may be done to monitor patients for heart damage. With proper supervision by experts familiar with the use of these drugs (medical oncologists), the risk of serious problems is small.

Cells in the ovaries of young women and cells in the testes of men are constantly dividing to produce ova (eggs) and spermatozoa (sperms) for potential reproduction. If chemo-therapy is essential in such people they are advised to avoid initiating a pregnancy during treatment and for at least 12 months afterwards due to the risk of producing abnormal ova or spermatozoa. There is even a risk of permanent sterility. In the case of men, semen can be collected and kept deep frozen in liquid nitrogen before chemotherapy is started. If needed, the semen can be used for *in vivo* or *in vitro* fertilisation at a later date. It may sometimes be possible to take and freeze ova from women before commencing chemotherapy. These can be fertilised and implanted into the uterus at a later date if subsequent cancer treatment has been successful. However, this procedure is still somewhat experimental.

Simultaneous chemo/radiotherapy

In treating locally advanced cancers with intra-arterial-induction chemotherapy, the intra-arterial infusion is given over a slow period of up to five weeks, with a break of three weeks before commencing radiotherapy. Provided this is closely monitored, it has been a very effective treatment for locally advanced cancers, such as those in the head and neck, breast and limbs. However, it is prolonged and expensive in length of hospital-bed occupation.

More recently, simultaneous chemotherapy and radiotherapy has achieved similar results in controlling locally advanced cancers. These treatment programs are simpler to deliver as the chemotherapy is given systemically. The chemotherapy sensitises the cancer cells, as well as other cells, to radiotherapy, making the local radiotherapy more effective. However, all cells in the radiation fields are made more sensitive to the radiotherapy, so not only is the cancer destroyed, so too may be any normal cells in the irradiated region. The doses of chemotherapy and radiotherapy are therefore even more critically balanced between being insufficient on the one hand, or on the other hand causing potentially dangerous damage to surrounding tissues such as nearby arteries. The safest but most effective combinations are still being studied in many situations.

OTHER IMPORTANT TREATMENTS

Hormone therapy

The first evidence that some cancers would respond to hormonal treatment was reported in 1886 in Scotland when a Dr Beatson reported regression of a breast cancer after removal of a woman's ovaries.

In 1941 two American doctors, Charles Huggins and Clarence Hodges, showed that in a large percentage of cases, cancers of the prostate regressed either after the removal of male hormone (by castration) or by the administration of a female hormone (oestrogen). These were the first indications that some cancers are hormone dependent and could respond to the manipulation of certain natural body hormones. Since then some other cancers have been found to be hormone dependent (e.g. cancer in the male breast). Often these hormonal influences can be reduced by giving the patient an antagonistic hormone. A cancer that is stimulated by or dependent on a particular type of hormone is likely to be inhibited or suppressed by the removal of the source of that hormone, or by giving a hormone that has the opposite effect. Today castration of males is rarely used as treatment because newer drugs, which either antagonise testosterone or prevent its synthesis, are available. These can be given as tablets orally or as pellet implants that last for some three months. These implant drugs are termed LH-RH antagonists, inhibiting the release of signal hormones from the pituitary gland (at the base of the brain), which stimulates testosterone production by the testis.

Breast cancer

In a number of women breast cancer is, to varying extents, dependent on the female hormone oestrogen. This dependency can be detected by testing for the presence of a protein called the oestrogen receptor. Giving more oestrogen to these patients could cause the cancer to grow more rapidly. On the other hand, removing the source of the patient's naturally produced oestrogen (removal of ovaries in pre-menopausal women) results in regression of the breast cancer to a greater or lesser degree in most patients. Removal of the ovaries can be used in treating cancer of the breast in younger women and as an adjuvant after surgery as well if the cancer is widespread. Unfortunately, removal of the ovaries and other hormone treatments rarely, if ever, result in complete cure but often result in worthwhile remission, which may even last for some years.

The anti-oestrogen drug tamoxifen is, however, more widely used than removal of the ovaries.

In older women whose ovaries are not actively functioning, or in younger women who have had their ovaries removed, remission may be achieved by giving a new class of drugs that prevent oestrogen production in tissues other than the ovaries. Such drugs are called peripheral aromatase inhibitors.

Although tamoxifen has been the most effective and most widely used anti-hormone, and rarely causes any upset to the patient in the short term (over a year or two), when used over several years there is some risk that it may alter and even stimulate a cancer in the uterus. This risk is quite small, but most doctors now limit the use of tamoxifen to about two to five years unless it is essential to use it for longer periods.

Manipulation of hormones, such as the use of tamoxifen, has a distinct advantage over other forms of chemotherapy as hormones are less likely to cause prolonged nausea or other serious side effects. The newer peripheral aromatase inhibitors, such as Femara or Arimidex, are even more effective than tamoxifen. They work in post-menopausal women by inhibiting residual oestrogen synthesis in the body, particularly in fat tissues. The LH-RH antagonists used in prostate cancer can also be used in treating metastatic breast cancer.

Not all breast cancers will respond to hormone therapy. When a breast cancer biopsy is taken, a small piece is usually tested for hormone sensitivity (called the oestrogen and progesterone receptor tests). These tests will give an indication as to whether the cancer is likely to respond to hormone manipulation. If not, then some other form of treatment, such as cytotoxic chemotherapy, may be used.

The adrenal-gland hormone cortisone may also have the effect of suppressing some cancers. It is often used in combination with cytotoxic chemotherapeutic drugs in the treatment of breast cancer; some cases of leukaemia; the lymphomas, especially Hodgkin disease; adenocarcinoma of the kidney; and a rare cancer of bone marrow called multiple myeloma. This type of cortisone-like drug is either dexamethasone or prednisone.

Prostate cancer

Prostate cancers are hormone dependent. Prostate cancer will not grow in the absence of androgen, the male hormone. Treatment of widespread prostate cancer with excess female hormones or anti-androgens is described in Section 3.

Other cancers that respond to hormones

These include cancer in the male breast, which will often respond to castration, and cancer of the lining inside the womb (endometrial cancer of the uterus), which may respond to the hormone progesterone. Very rarely cancer of the kidney will respond to the female hormone progesterone, and occasionally thyroid cancer will be suppressed by the use of the thyroid hormone thyroxin.

Hormone side effects

Hormone therapy has the advantage of being well tolerated by most patients and relatively free of serious side effects in comparison to cytotoxic chemotherapeutic drugs. However, hormones may sometimes have some side effects, generally mimicking menopause-like symptoms in women.

Hormone treatment is often accepted by patients and the medical profession as being more natural, more scientific and less toxic than cytotoxic chemotherapy. Unfortunately, however, the good responses of hormone treatment are not permanent in patients with metastatic disease, and almost invariably the cancers relapse after some months or years. Each time they redevelop they are less responsive to other forms of hormone management and eventually become unaffected by all forms of hormone management.

Immunotherapy

The body's natural defence against invasion by organisms and other foreign matter is through its immune system. There is some evidence that the body also has immune defences against malignant cells, and the development of certain cancers is possibly due to some defect in these protective mechanisms.

Much research is concerned with determining the nature of these immunological defence mechanisms and trying to improve or assist them. The most striking breakthrough has been the development of certain 'monoclonal antibodies' that are often effective, such as Herceptin in breast cancer, Mabthera in lymphoma and Erbitux in bowel cancer (see below).

Some years ago injections of certain relatively harmless organisms such as the cowpox virus, BCG (a harmless bacterium) or Corynebacterium parvum (another harmless bacterium) were used in trials in the treatment of some malignancies to stimulate natural immune defence mechanisms. Some isolated successes were reported with these and other 'immune' preparations, especially in the treatment of melanoma and lymphomas, but as yet consistent clinical benefit has not been found and for most cancers little if any benefit has resulted. The most effective application of BCG now in use is in treatment of some bladder cancers.

New immune preparations are constantly under study, but three groups of immunological substances of particular interest are the interferons, the interleukins and tumour necrosis factor (TNF).

Interferon

It was first recognised in the 1930s that infection of animal cells with one virus would, for a time, 'interfere' with infection by other viruses. Thirty years later it was discovered that a protein substance was released from cells infected with a virus, and this substance protected other cells against other viral infections. This interfering substance is called interferon.

Interferon is species specific. That is, interferon produced by chicken cells is protective of other chicken cells against virus infection but does not give similar protection in any other animal. Similarly, interferon produced from human cells is protective for other human cells but not for cells of other animal species. Interferon is now manufactured by recombinant DNA technology and is available for clinical use. It can be quite toxic, causing lassitude and flu-like symptoms. It is sometimes used after surgery for melanoma and in some patients with metastatic renal cancer, certain lymphomas and myeloma.

The condition AIDS is caused by virus infection. This condition is an infection and not a cancer, but it can result in the development of a particular type of cancer called Kaposi's sarcoma and virulent forms of lymphoma. However, the use of powerful antiviral drug treatment in AIDS patients has now prevented most of these cancers from occurring.

The interleukins

The interleukins are protein substances produced from white cells and are found to activate the immunological defence system. The first interleukins were Interleukin I, which is produced from macrophages (giant white cells) and Interleukin II, which is produced from lymphocytes (small white cells). They stimulate reproduction and activity of immune cells against a cancer to which the cells have been specifically sensitised. In experimental animals, interleukins have been shown under certain conditions to so stimulate the animal's natural lymphocyte activity against implanted cancers that the cancers have been completely eradicated. However, at the time of writing, neither Interleukin I nor Interleukin II nor several more recently discovered interleukins have made any major impact on cancer treatment.

Tumour-necrosis factor (TNF)

TNF is a more recent product of immunological research. This product does cause cancer-cell destruction in some experimental models but is too toxic for direct use in human patients. Recent work in Europe has shown, however, that TNF enhances the anti-cancer effect of certain other anti-cancer agents and can be used safely and effectively when given to a part of the body only. At the time of writing it can only be safely given in a closed circuit by regional perfusion or regional infusion to treat malignancies such as melanoma and sarcoma when confined to a limb (see 'Regional chemotherapy' above).

Monoclonal antibodies

Recently developed techniques in biotechnology have made it possible to manufacture so-called monoclonal antibodies that are aimed at specific vital targets in certain cancers. These include malignant lymphoma, breast and bowel cancers. The use of these antibodies is relatively new (e.g. Mabthera for lymphoma, Herceptin in breast cancer and Erbitux for bowel cancer). In general these antibodies are used in combination with chemotherapy. Despite their great expense they are showing considerable effectiveness, although their final role is still being evaluated.

Small-molecule target inhibitors

Basic cancer research has lead to a detailed understanding of how growth-signalling cytokines circulate in the blood and bind to cancer cells via special receptor molecules. These receptors become activated by the binding cytokine and send a complex series of chemical signals to the cell nucleus, stimulating cell growth and division. The inhibitors prevent this happening so that cell division is impaired.

SOME TREATMENTS UNDER STUDY

Heat therapy

It is well known that cancer cells are more sensitive to heat than normal cells. A number of researchers and clinicians have been investigating methods of applying localised heat to organs or tissues containing cancer in a manner that will safely destroy the cancer cells but not damage the normal body tissues. This approach could be particularly valuable for treating cancer cells in vital organs that cannot be safely removed, such as the liver. Several types of microwave-emitting machines have been designed for this purpose. A number of problems have yet to be solved, particularly in maintaining the heat at a critical level for a significant period without overheating the patient or causing damage to normal tissues and cells. After several years of study the most that can be said is that some interesting and hopeful results have been reported.

Heat therapy is also being studied in conjunction with chemotherapy in treating some cancers confined to a limb (e.g. melanoma). There is no doubt that when the chemotherapy and heat can be confined to the limb circulation there is a greater cancer response than when chemotherapy alone is used. However, with this combined treatment there is also more risk of damage to normal muscles, skin and other tissues in the limb.

Laser surgery

Laser surgery is simply a development of surgical technique in cancer treatment in which a laser is used to cut or destroy cancer tissue that is exposed to the laser light. Laser treatment is showing some promise in treating early cancers of the prostate.

Cryosurgery

This is a technique of destroying cancer tissue by using an extremely cold temperature application to freeze it. When the application is removed, the frozen crystallised tissue naturally returns to body temperature, causing the cancer cells to fragment and die. This process is known as 'freeze–thaw'. It has been used for years to treat small pre-malignant skin lesions (using dry ice or liquid nitrogen), but recently probes have been developed to destroy secondary deposits of cancer cells, especially in the liver.

Photodynamic therapy

Photodynamic therapy is a relatively new type of treatment being investigated for some cancers.

The new capillary blood vessels that develop with a cancer to supply it with blood are small, poorly formed and fragile. They easily break down if damaged and also allow some chemicals to leak out into the cancer tissues. Photodynamic therapy depends on a technique of giving the patients certain photosensitive chemical substances by intravenous injection. These substances leak out of the fragile blood vessels in the cancer and the cancer is then subjected to laser light of certain wavelengths. The reaction of the substances to laser light destroys the cancer cells. As laser light does not penetrate any distance into tissues, this treatment is only used at this stage to treat certain surface cancers such as those in the skin or in the mucous membrane lining the mouth. Studies to date are being carried out only in highly specialised clinics as precautions must be taken to avoid side effects, especially general sunlight hypersensitivity.

The advantages of this treatment over other more standard treatments are as yet uncertain, but in the future there may be potential for developing similar techniques to treat other less accessible cancers.

Anti-angiogenesis

Following the principles mentioned in photodynamic therapy, agents are now being developed that are specifically aimed at damaging or preventing development of the small blood vessels (capillaries) that supply the cancers with blood. Without a blood supply the cancers can't grow or survive. At this stage successful experiments have been conducted against cancers in mice and other animals. One such product is called 'angiostatin', but it is likely that a number of new agents, aimed specifically at cancer blood vessels, will be developed in the near future.

People who remember the deformed limbs of babies born in the early 1960s to some mothers who took the anti-nausea drug thalidomide may be interested to know that thalidomide caused the defects precisely as a result of interfering with the important blood vessels growing in the developing foetus limbs at a crucial time of foetal development. Thalidomide and similar products are now being investigated to destroy the small blood vessels in some growing cancers.

Watch this space!

GENERAL HEALTHCARE IN PATIENTS WITH CANCER

The presence of advancing cancer in the body will sooner or later have a profound effect on the patient's general state of health. Anorexia (loss of appetite), weight loss, anaemia, lassitude and general debility are common general features, and specific problems will develop according to the site of the cancer and the tissues or organs involved. The ability of the body's natural defence mechanisms to control cancer will be affected by the patient's general state of health, mental and emotional state and ability to tolerate the various forms of treatment.

For these reasons it is important that special attention be paid to the patient's general health. His or her diet should be nutritious yet tempting and interesting. Adequate vitamins must be provided either in the food or with vitamin supplements. Any anaemia should be appropriately treated, and there should be provision for adequate rest and gentle healthy exercise. There must also be adequate provision for pain relief.

TREATMENT OF COMPLICATIONS AND PALLIATIVE CARE

Special problems associated with particular forms of cancer will need appropriate care. This may include attention to nutrition for patients with obstructive cancer of the oesophagus or stomach; relief of obstruction for patients with bowel cancer causing bowel obstruction or pancreatic cancer causing bile-duct obstruction and jaundice; relief of urinary obstruction in cancer of the prostate gland; and adequate local treatment and dressing for cancers fungating through the skin. Pressure on the lungs with breathlessness caused by fluid accumulated around the lungs in the pleural cavity (hydrothorax) may be at least temporarily relieved by removing the fluid. Similarly, removal of fluid accumulated in the abdominal cavity (ascites) may temporarily relieve pressure in the abdomen and lower chest (paracentesis).

Raised intra-cranial pressure (inside the skull) may cause headaches, vomiting, convulsions or loss of consciousness (coma). This may be caused by cancers with surrounding swelling in the brain. The patient can often be relieved by the use of cortisone-like drugs to reduce the swelling or by radiotherapy.

Complicating infections with cancer, such as pneumonia associated with cancer obstructing the air passages, will also require appropriate attention.

Bones involved with cancer may not only be painful but may fracture spontaneously, a condition known as pathological fracture. Pathological fractures need to be treated on their merits (e.g. with surgical pinning), but healing is often helped by local radiotherapy. Newer drugs called bisphosphonates are often given to patients at high risk of developing bone metastases, especially those with breast or prostate cancer, as well as multiple myeloma. Secondary cancers in the liver, lungs, brain, bowel and other locations may also need special treatment.

PAIN RELIEF

Nothing is more wearing, debilitating and distressing for people than to suffer constant pain. Although most cancers causing severe pain are usually advanced and some are not curable, patients suffering from severe pain can at least be given relief. For curable cancers the best pain relief is achieved by eradicating the cancer, but many new pain-relieving measures are available for incurable cancers. Radiotherapy will often reduce the size of the cancer and reduce surrounding swelling and pressure, so giving pain relief. This is especially true for secondary cancers in bones and the brain. Operations to relieve obstruction of bowel, bladder or other organs will give pain relief. Hormones or anti-cancer drugs that reduce the size of cancers, thus reducing any associated pressure, may also be used on occasions to effect pain relief.

Nerves that transmit pain sensation may also be put out of action by injecting them with local anaesthetic or with alcohol or, rarely, by cutting them surgically to relieve pain. Occasionally the nerve pathway in the spinal cord that conducts pain sensation to the brain can be cut to give permanent loss of pain sensation from a region of the body.

Meditation, hypnotherapy or acupuncture are sometimes used for pain relief. Although these may be helpful with some patients, with others their greatest value may be in emotional support rather than in relief of severe or constant pain.

Pain-relieving drugs are the most common and quickest method of pain relief, either simple pain-relieving drugs (analgesics) or stronger and addictive pain-relieving drugs (narcotics). Simple analgesics such as aspirin and aspirin-like products, paracetamol (acetaminophen) and the like are usually used first. If these are not effective, agents containing small amounts of the least dangerous narcotic agent, codeine, are often used. Stronger narcotic agents such as morphine may be given when specific anti-cancer treatments are ineffective. There are slow-release oral preparations of morphine and related drugs that are simple for patients to use, avoiding frequent injections. They are given once or twice a day for as long as necessary. Alternatively, small pumps can be used to give morphine by subcutaneous infusion. These are available for home use and managed by palliative care nurses who do home visits as required. A disadvantage of morphine is nausea in some patients and constipation in most. Careful use of laxatives is always necessary. In some countries heroin is also used very effectively in these circumstances, but only where it is certain that life expectancy is strictly limited. There are also analgesic drugs as effective as morphine that can be given by a 'patch' (e.g. Durogesic) attached to the skin. These patches can provide good pain relief for up to three days. They also have the advantage of not causing constipation.

PSYCHOTHERAPY AND SPIRITUAL HELP

Some psychologists and alternative-medicine practitioners, as well as some psychiatrists, postulate that sometimes cancer may be a result of anxiety, psychological trauma or depressive states. There is little hard evidence for this. However, it must be recognised that certain emotional states may well be detrimental to a patient's wellbeing with an adverse effect on the disease and response to treatment. This is a natural and understandable reaction to what was previously regarded as a death sentence at worst, or at best a serious illness requiring radical or prolonged treatment and possibly disfigurement.

Such emotional distress will often cause patients to seek alternative or fringe-medicine therapists, especially if they have been told that mainstream medicine has little to offer.

These natural reactions should be anticipated by all doctors who care for cancer patients. Support for the emotional needs of the patient and the patient's family should be readily available in all situations. Such support can be given most effectively by the responsible clinicians in concert with the multidisciplinary cancer treatment team. The participation of a psychiatrist or psychologist experienced in this field with the cancer-treatment team can be invaluable.

Some have claimed that some patients who have learned techniques of relaxation, meditation or hypnotherapy have shown not only emotional and physical benefit but even regressions of their cancer. In some traditions acupuncture has given similar benefit. Such benefits are difficult to evaluate, as cases of spontaneous cancer regression have been reported in the medical literature. However, an experienced psychiatrist, clinical psychologist or social worker can help the cancer patient and members of his or her family adjust to the new situation and its associated emotional, social and other problems. A social worker can advise on various agency supports that may be available. For many people, especially those with advanced or incurable cancer, an experienced member of the clergy or other spiritual advisor can be invaluable.

PALLIATIVE CARE

In recent years doctors, nurses and paramedical workers have developed a new specialty in palliative care. These specialists have now become most valuable members of cancer-treatment teams. They are expert in sophisticated measures used to control pain and other potentially distressing symptoms. They have links with the domiciliary nursing-care teams and in-patient hospice units. They can significantly help both patients and their families adjust to difficult circumstances and needs in the terminal phase of cancer.

FOLLOW-UP CARE

No matter what treatments have been used, it is important for patients to have regular follow-up medical examinations. The purpose of these is to detect and treat any recurring problem at an early stage. If no evidence of residual disease is detected, it gives patients confidence that their disease has been cured or at least continues in remission.

It is also important for doctors to keep records to document the outcome of various new treatment approaches that are being increasingly developed in the form of clinical trials. In general if a patient's disease has not recurred within five years after treatment, it is highly likely that the patient is cured. However, such individuals should realise that they, like anyone else, remain at risk of other diseases, including cancers of a different type.

Two of the more common cancers, however, require a longer period of regular follow-up, as the disease may reoccur many years later. These are melanoma and breast cancer. It seems the body's natural immune defences can keep these cancers under control for many years until something causes it to recur. These recurrences are often slow growing and may be curable if they have been detected while still small and localised, hence the special need for continued follow-up of these patients.

UNORTHODOX AND FRINGE MEDICINE

Until a century or two ago all medical treatments were somewhat speculative, based on one-off observations, traditions, 'old wives' tales', naturopathic practices, herbs or other unsourced or specifically unproven remedies.

There are still almost limitless numbers of 'cancer cures' promoted by a variety of people ranging from well-intentioned unorthodox or fringe medical practitioners on the one hand to misguided quacks and unscrupulous charlatans on the other.

These 'cancer cures' range from large doses of vitamins (especially vitamin C, vitamin E and other antioxidants) to preparations of herbs, a variety of plant extracts (one of the most publicised being an extract of apricot kernels, laetrile), diets (especially low-protein diets), to meditation, acupuncture, hypnotherapy and faith healing. At the other extreme are sleight-of-hand manoeuvres in which practitioners pretend to extract cancers painlessly.

Some of these so-called cures may be based on coincidental observation of a cancer patient who happened to undergo a spontaneous remission rather than on scientific knowledge. Such remissions (though extremely rare) are well recorded in cases such as osteogenic sarcoma, renal cancer and melanoma.

In general alternative-medicine 'cures' have been investigated and found to be without basis. Patients who find themselves unable to face the reality of an incurable condition or radical surgery will often search for a more acceptable alternative. This is understandable and must be appreciated by cancer-treatment teams, who must be prepared to spend time in advising and helping cancer patients in their emotional as well as their physical distress.

At the same time doctors should not close their minds to ideas proposed by unorthodox practitioners that may later be of value in cancer treatment. Most such proposed cancer cures undergo assessment by appropriate authorities.

For some patients certain alternative therapies can be very comforting and supportive, even though they are essentially an emotional or psychological crutch. Often patients feel such therapies are offering them a more active role in coping with their disease. Provided such therapy is not harmful either physically or financially, and does not conflict with appropriate treatment, it can be supported by the cancer therapy team.

LEGALISING VOLUNTARY EUTHANASIA

Voluntary euthanasia has been the subject of passionate debate. It is not appropriate to attempt in this book to resolve the many issues that have been raised.

In Australia people who promote euthanasia do so to allow those who are believed to be suffering from prolonged pain and distress to end their lives with dignity. This would occur after assessment by independent qualified doctors who have agreed that there is no reasonable alternative.

On the other hand, many people oppose euthanasia. Some oppose it on the basis of strongly held religious convictions, but others express reservations for many reasons, including the following:

- High standards of palliative care are freely available in most developed countries, including Australia. Such care can allow a valuable period of good life quality to people previously experiencing severe pain or other distressing symptoms.

- Appropriate access to pain-relieving medication, including narcotics, is widely available. The law clearly notes that narcotic medication given with the primary intent to relieve symptoms is appropriate, even though this may shorten life by a small amount.

- Individuals have the right to refuse artificial means of keeping alive family members or themselves if they are in an otherwise terminal situation. Doctors are likewise discouraged from giving blood transfusions or other treatments to patients to inappropriately prolong life.

- Some people who have a depressive illness may develop another disease such as cancer. They may use such a diagnosis to request help in what is essentially suicide. Not all patients, even those with advanced cancer, are prepared to acknowledge the benefits of pain-relieving drugs or other good palliative care when they wish to end their lives for other reasons.

- Many doctors, nurses and other health professionals are unhappy that the highest ideals of their professions could become compromised if the role of 'takers of human life' were delegated to them. They see their role as being quite different and would prefer to be viewed as people whom patients can trust to preserve their lives with as little pain or distress as is possible.

Perhaps the greatest worry of all to most medical practitioners is that no matter where a line is drawn, there would always be exceptions that at first appear reasonable. Gradually the laws would be compromised, leading to abuse or inappropriate use of euthanasia should it be a formal legal option.

3
Some common cancers

SKIN CANCERS

Cancer of the skin most commonly affects people of fair-skinned northern European descent in regions closer to the equator, such as Australia. Australians have the world's highest incidence of skin cancer, followed by the white populations of the southern regions of the USA.

There are three basic types of skin cancer: basal-cell carcinoma (BCC), which is by far the most common and, fortunately, the least dangerous; squamous-cell carcinoma (SCC), which is the next most frequent; and melanoma, which is much rarer but the most dangerous.

BCC

A BCC is usually first noticed as a small crusty patch, nodule or ulcer. These cancers occur most commonly in skin that has been constantly exposed to sunshine over many years. Hence they are not common before the age of 40 and become more frequent with increasing age. More than 70% of these cancers occur on the face, as it is most constantly exposed to the sun. The next most common sites are the neck, the backs of the hands or forearms, the lower legs, chest and back.

BCCs are not painful and are usually slow growing; patients may have noticed them for months or even years before they seek medical attention. If neglected, they usually develop as slowly enlarging ulcers (sometimes called 'rodent' ulcers because they may look like skin that has been gnawed by a rodent). Although, fortunately, they almost never spread to lymph nodes or other distant tissues, they do tend to erode locally into tissues around them. If neglected for a long time, they may become incurable or even fatal by causing destruction to such tissues as underlying cartilage of the nose or ear, the underlying bone of the skull or large blood vessels in the neck. They can sometimes invade the orbit and paranasal sinuses and may even erode into the brain.

Treatment

BCCs can be easily and effectively cured in their early stages by simple surgical excision, usually under local anaesthesia. The specimen of tissue excised is examined under a microscope by a pathologist to confirm that it was a BCC and that it was completely excised with an adequate margin of normal tissue. Radiotherapy is also an effective method of treating many BCCs but preferably after a small biopsy has been taken to confirm the diagnosis. Radiotherapy has the advantage of avoiding surgical operation and being a painless procedure; it has the disadvantage of requiring expensive specialised equipment and personnel and several treatment attendances, and it leaves some permanent damage to a small patch of skin. Another disadvantage is that if no tissue is removed, there may be some doubt about the exact diagnosis of the lesion and whether it was completely eradicated. However, for many small lesions, especially in elderly patients, it may be the most appropriate form of treatment.

Sometimes small BCCs are removed by dermatologists (skin specialists) using cauterisation or a small curette (a scraping instrument). These techniques should be left to experienced experts, as a mistake in diagnosis or incomplete removal can lead to a greater problem.

BCCs that recur after previous failed attempts at treatment, or those occurring close to vital structures such as a tear duct or an eyelid, present special problems and require expert attention.

Large BCCs invading bone or other tissues may require extensive surgical procedures, including reconstructive surgery. Occasionally they may even be incurable and are possibly best treated by palliative radiotherapy. (Palliative treatment will give a patient relief by reducing the cancer or lessening its symptoms, without being likely to cure it.)

Although such advanced lesions are rare, they are disastrous when they do occur and can easily be prevented by correct treatment in their early stages. Hence the importance of people with small lesions seeking medical help early when BCCs are easily and completely curable.

SCC

SCCs are also most common on the skin of the face, especially the lower part of the face and lower lip, but they also often occur on the neck, the backs of the hands or forearms and the skin of other frequently exposed areas such as the legs, back or chest. People who have had kidney transplants are at high risk for frequent and recurrent SCCs because of the immunosuppressive treatment they receive.

SCCs often develop in skin lesions called hyperkeratoses, which are small, crusty or flaky thickened areas of skin resulting from previous longstanding sun damage.

An SCC is usually first noticed as a small, painless lump growing on the skin's surface or as an ulcer in the skin. SCCs usually grow more rapidly than BCCs and after a time tend to spread to nearby draining lymph nodes. Later, they may spread further to more distant lymph nodes or even to other distant tissues or organs such as the lung. They also grow locally and are likely to invade surrounding tissues that may ulcerate, bleed and become painful.

Fortunately, most SCCs of the skin have not spread when they are first diagnosed, and treatment of the draining lymph nodes is usually not required. However, the draining lymph nodes must be kept under close observation and in case of enlargement should be treated without delay, usually by surgical excision.

Treatment

As for all cancers, the earlier these lesions are diagnosed and treated, the less radical the treatment they need and the greater the likelihood of cure.

For any lesion suspected of being an SCC, it is important to obtain a tissue diagnosis; that is, for a biopsy to be taken. In the case of a small lesion, this may be best achieved by surgical excision of the whole lesion (an excision biopsy). For a large lesion it is usually more appropriate for a small piece of tissue to be taken from its edge for biopsy and microscopic examination (an incision biopsy). A frozen-section examination of a biopsy specimen, as described in Section 2, may be appropriate to allow complete treatment to be carried out without delay.

Once the diagnosis of an SCC is established, treatment is by surgical excision or sometimes by radiotherapy. Surgical excision is usually the most effective and most appropriate treatment. The lesion is widely excised and examined microscopically to confirm that a margin of normal tissue surrounding the cancer has also been excised, ensuring that removal of all the primary cancer has been achieved. If the draining lymph nodes are enlarged, without evidence that this is due to infection, the lymph nodes should also be removed, in one block of tissue. Depending on the site and how much tissue has to be excised, a plastic surgical procedure such as a skin graft may be needed to repair the tissue and close the wound.

As in the case of BCCs, radiotherapy may be used to treat some SCCs of the skin, especially in elderly patients, in cases where an operation might be risky or occasionally as palliative treatment when cure by surgery is not possible.

Occasionally when an SCC of skin is very advanced or invading vital organs or other tissues, or when it has become incurable by local surgery because of secondary spread, it may be appropriate to use anti-cancer drugs to reduce the extent and size of the cancer and to relieve symptoms. Large SCCs of the skin sometimes appear incurable by radiotherapy or surgery (or only curable by mutilating surgery such as amputation of a limb). These can occasionally be reduced in size and extent by chemotherapy first, especially when given regionally by intra-arterial infusion (as described in Section 2). After chemotherapy the cancers are often so reduced in size, extent and viability that they can be cured by radiotherapy and/or local surgical excision.

Melanoma

Melanoma, the most dangerous form of skin cancer, is a malignant growth of pigment-forming cells in skin or the eye. Occasionally they may occur in mucous membranes such as the lining of the mouth or anus.

Although melanoma is a highly malignant tumour, present-day management methods have greatly improved the outlook. Considered to be incurable in about 50% of patients 50 years ago, melanoma in Australia, where it is usually diagnosed early, is now cured in more than 90% of cases.

The exact cause of melanoma is not known, although it is most common in fair-skinned people living in sunny tropical or subtropical climates. Unlike BCCs and SCCs, however, melanoma is not more common on the areas of the body most constantly exposed to sunshine. The most common sites are on the backs of men and the thighs of women. However, in common with other skin cancers, the world's highest incidence of melanoma is in the white population of Australia, especially those living closest to the equator and nearest to the seaside. The white population of the sunny southern parts of the USA also has a high incidence of melanoma. People of dark-skinned races do occasionally develop a melanoma, but in these people it is more commonly at sites of less pigmentation, such as the sole of the foot, under fingernails or toenails or in the mucosal lining of the mouth or anus.

Melanoma rarely affects children before puberty. After puberty it can affect people of any age, including teenagers and young adults as well as middle-aged and older people. Melanoma is now more common in men, and the survival rate for women is better.

The danger of melanoma lies in the fact that it can spread relatively early to draining lymph nodes and to distant organs such as the liver, lungs, bowel wall and brain. The outlook has improved because people in general, and doctors in particular, are more aware of the early features of melanoma and the need to commence treatment as early as possible. Most melanomas develop in pre-existing moles in the skin, but others develop in areas of unaffected skin. Occasionally a melanoma will develop without pigment. This is known as an amelanotic melanoma and can be diagnosed only by microscopic examination. Amelanotic melanomas behave in a similar way to pigmented melanomas and require similar treatment.

Symptoms and signs

Any evidence of increasing pigmentation in a spot in the skin, or an increase in size or pigmentation of a mole, must be regarded with suspicion. Other early features may be itching or crusting of a mole. Bleeding and ulceration are usually later features. Any of these features occurring either in a pre-existing mole or in a newly pigmented spot require immediate attention, and if there is any doubt an excision biopsy should be done.

Treatment

Surgical excision of early lesions offers the best hope of cure. Early melanomas can be excised with generally a 1 cm margin of normal surrounding tissue as their cells are sometimes present in tissues or even in lymphatic vessels surrounding the cancer. Thicker, crusted or bleeding melanomas require a wider margin. If there is evidence of draining-lymph-node involvement, then these lymph nodes should also be excised in one block of tissue.

The likelihood of the melanoma spreading is directly related to the thickness (depth) of the malignant cells, so that in the case of thick lesions, a sentinel-lymph-node biopsy may be performed. This is similar to the procedure performed in breast cancer. A dye or radio-tracer is injected into the skin near the melanoma. This allows discovery and removal of the first draining 'sentinel' node or nodes. This node (or sometimes two or three nodes) is then examined microscopically by the pathologist. If it is involved with metastatic disease, the remaining nodes in that group are also surgically removed.

Melanomas are not particularly sensitive to radiotherapy, although radiotherapy may be helpful in some situations such as for a secondary melanoma in the brain. They are also generally resistant to chemotherapy.

When advanced melanoma appears to be confined to one limb, treatment by more concentrated regional chemotherapy, via a special technique into the blood supply of that limb only, often achieves worthwhile improvement, with cancer regression. This technique is called 'closed circuit' or isolation perfusion. A newer, more easily used technique is 'closed circuit infusion'. This treatment is more effective if heat is used with the chemotherapy and appears to be even more effective if the new immunotherapy agent TNF (tumour necrosis factor) is used with chemotherapy.

Immunotherapy is also sometimes used in the treatment of advanced or widespread melanoma. Although some improvements have been observed with general (systemic) immunotherapy, most results have been inconsistent, and early hopes of a reliable new cure have not yet been fulfilled. In some patients with lymph-node involvement, a high dose of interferon is given to try to prevent recurrence, but side effects may make this quite difficult for the patient to cope with.

Trials with chemotherapy and immunotherapy are ongoing in melanoma clinics in the hope of improving outcomes for patients with more advanced stages of disease.

LUNG CANCER

Cancer of the lung, a relatively rare disease prior to World War I, now causes more deaths in males than any other cancer. It will soon overtake breast cancer as the main cause of cancer death in women. These rapid increases in incidence are directly related to cigarette smoking. The disease is ten to 20 times more common in smokers than in non-smokers.

Although tobacco smoking is by far the most significant cause, a number of other factors may also play a part in some cases, including industrial and automobile pollutant gases. Workers in certain industries, including the chromium, arsenic and asbestos industries, may have an additional increased incidence, especially if they are smokers.

Symptoms and signs

In its early stages lung cancer usually causes no noticeable new symptoms, so it is often diagnosed at an advanced stage when it is incurable. This may be due to lack of recognition of an increasing cough in heavy smokers who have had a cough for years. Other than a cough the common symptoms are blood-stained sputum, chest pain and episodes of chest infection or pneumonia, which do not completely resolve after treatment with antibiotics.

The first signs of lung cancer may also be evidence of metastatic spread to lymph nodes, bone, brain or elsewhere. In rare cases lung cancers produce hormone-like substances that may result in changes to other parts of the body such as swelling of the breasts, changes in bones, fingernails (clubbing) or loss of various brain or nerve functions.

Investigations

By the time symptoms are present, a chest X-ray will almost always reveal the cancer, but chest X-rays done for some other reason will sometimes show a lung cancer that has not been causing symptoms.

CT scans will show more clearly the position and size of a lung cancer in relation to other structures.

Bronchoscopy (examination of the air passages with a bronchoscope) will often allow the doctor to see a tumour in the larger airways (bronchi). A biopsy of the suspected cancer may be taken and examined under a microscope to confirm that cancer is present, to find out what sort of lung cancer it is and therefore how best to treat it.

Sometimes a cancer cannot be seen through a bronchoscope but can be detected in sputum that has been aspirated (sucked out) or coughed up and examined under a microscope. This test is called cytology. It will often show cancer cells if a cancer is present. If a lump is seen on X-ray, sometimes it is possible to aspirate cells for cytology from the lump through a needle inserted through the chest wall (see Section 2).

Treatment

A major advance has been the application of PET scanning (see Section 2). This has improved the ability of doctors to determine whether a lung cancer is operable or not. As well as the actual primary cancer any cancer extension or metastases will take up the radio-isotope labelled tracer. In many patients this test will avoid a futile operation where the chest is surgically opened and an unremovable cancer discovered. However, for those patients with localised disease, surgical resection offers the best chance of cure. PET scanning can also better define the exact extent of inoperable cancers to allow intensive local radiotherapy to begin without delay in some patients. A number of these patients can experience long-term remission with this approach. In some patients it is necessary to follow up lung-resection surgery with a combination of chemotherapy and radiotherapy: adjuvant therapy. Palliative chemotherapy for inoperable or metastatic lung cancer has improved with the new types of drugs that have become available in the last few years. Remissions, with improved quality of life, may last for several months.

Mesothelioma

Mesothelioma is a rare form of cancer occurring usually in people who have been exposed to asbestos either at work (e.g. in the construction and insulation industry or in the manufacture of asbestos products) or in home renovations. Mesothelioma is a malignancy of the tissues surrounding and lining the lungs (the pleura). It may also commence in the lining of the abdominal cavity (the peritoneum).

Symptoms

Mesothelioma patients may seek treatment for a cough, chest infection, difficulty with breathing or chest pain and a general feeling of being unwell and without energy.

Signs

Patients first consulting with mesothelioma often look pale, thin and with decreased movement of the chest and distressed breathing. They may be found to have a cancer or fluid collection around the lungs. The fluid collection may be seen on an X-ray or CT scan.

Mesothelioma is almost always fatal, as it is usually too widespread to treat by surgery. However, in some patients with relatively limited disease surgical removal of any obvious cancer mass may improve survival. The accumulations of fluid in the chest cavity can often be controlled by a pleurodesis, that is a procedure that causes the lung lining to adhere to the chest wall lining by injection of a special form of talc powder into the chest cavity. This procedure obliterates the pleural cavity around the lung so that fluid can't collect there and press on the lungs. Newer forms of chemotherapy can also achieve remissions lasting several months. Obviously, expert palliative care is critical to reduce symptoms to a minimum.

Secondary (metastatic) cancer involving the lung

Other than the nearby lymph nodes, the lungs (together with the liver) are the commonest sites of metastatic cancer. Cancers from almost any primary site can spread through the bloodstream to the lungs, e.g. from cancers of the breast, bowel, lung, kidney, testis, bone and melanoma of skin. Shortness of breath (dyspnoea) or cough are the main symptoms. Secondary cancers in the lungs usually show as a number of rounded opacities (white spots) on chest X-rays, although sometimes a secondary (especially from the kidney) may be single, showing as just one round white spot on an X-ray. Treatment depends on the type of primary cancer that has spread to the lung. Patients may respond to the specific forms of chemotherapy known to be effective for the primary-site cancer. For most cancer types this treatment will only be palliative, but sometimes, for some cancers, a cure is possible, especially with testicular cancer or lymphoma. For some patients with a limited number of metastases, surgical removal may be appropriate, and this may be curative (e.g. occasionally with melanoma, renal, testicular and bowel cancer, and bone and soft-tissue sarcomas). In metastatic breast or prostate cancer good remissions are sometimes possible with hormonal treatments (see Section 2).

Commonly, primary or secondary cancer in the lung will cause fluid to collect around the lung in the pleural cavity. This is known as a pleural effusion. This fluid can accumulate to the extent of several litres, causing shortness of breath as a result of pressure on the lung. Patients will get good relief following removal of this fluid with a simple drain tube or aspirating needle. This is often done in the X-ray department with ultrasound guidance. Talc-powder pleurodesis is commonly done in patients with recurrent effusions (see 'Mesothelioma' earlier).

BREAST CANCER

Breast cancer is now the most common cancer affecting women in Europe, the USA and Australia (excluding skin cancers). About one in ten Australian women will develop breast cancer during their lifetime. Although it is occasionally seen in younger women, breast cancer is not common until after the age of 40. The incidence then increases with age. The average age for women first presenting with breast cancer is about 60 years.

Although a specific cause of breast cancer is not known, there are a number of contributory factors. A highly significant factor is the age of a woman when she has her first child. Having a baby at an early age seems to give some protection, as breast cancer is least common in women who had their first babies as teenagers. It is more common in women who did not have their first baby until after the age of 30 or 35 years. This social phenomenon is one of the explanations for the increasing incidence of breast cancer in recent years. Women who have not had children are at greater risk from breast cancer.

The age at onset of menstruation and the age at menopause are also significant. Early menstruation and late menopause are both associated with an increased risk of breast cancer. Again these are related to improved modern Western standards of living. It seems that the greater number of years the woman's reproductive function continues, reflecting continuous exposure to the female sex hormone oestrogen, the greater the risk of breast cancer.

There may also be some protection in breastfeeding, although the evidence for this is less clear. This may be a result of reduction in oestrogen synthesis at this time.

There is an association between breast cancer and Western lifestyle factors such as a diet high in animal fat, obesity and alcohol, although these associations are not as clear as they are for tobacco smoking and lung cancer.

Breast injury is not known to cause breast cancer. Although some women first notice a lump after an injury that is in fact breast cancer, it is likely that in most cases the injury simply drew attention to the cancer that was already present. Injuries may, of course, cause other types of lumps in the breast that are not cancer.

Hormone-replacement therapy (HRT) has been suspected of increasing the risk of breast cancer. However, unless the woman had previously been treated for breast cancer or has some special risk factor (such as a strong family history of breast cancer), the risk of the small doses of hormones in HRT is small.

Nevertheless, for this reason, HRT is not given to every woman who reaches the menopause. For those with severe menopausal symptoms the improvement in quality of life may justify the small increased risk, provided the woman is kept under regular observation. Meanwhile, studies continue to try to find other forms of risk-free therapy to relieve these symptoms. One study is investigating the use of phytoestrogens that occur naturally in soybeans and other plant foods.

Cancer in the male breast does occur but at a rate of about 1% of that occurring in women. Such cancers behave in a similar way to cancer in female breasts. The approach to treatment is similar to that in women, with a similar outcome. A problem, however, is often a delay in diagnosis.

Symptoms and signs

Breast cancer is usually first noticed when a woman finds a painless lump in the breast. The most common location is in the upper outer part of the breast, and the lump is often first felt in the bath or shower when fingers are soapy and lumps are more easily felt.

By far the majority of breast lumps are not cancer. However, when a woman first notices a lump in a breast, she should have it examined by a doctor. If necessary, the woman should be sent for further investigation or for a specialist opinion.

Other features of breast cancer may be a change in the position or shape of a nipple (called retraction or inversion); puckering or ulceration of skin over the breast, especially if over a lump; discharge of blood from a nipple or discharge of other fluid from a nipple not associated with a pregnancy or lactation; redness of a nipple; or a change in the size of one breast. Occasionally the first indication of breast cancer is a red inflamed breast resembling breast infection (acute mastitis). If an acute mastitis develops for no apparent reason or does not settle down with appropriate treatment (including antibiotics), the possibility of an underlying cancer must be considered.

Sometimes breast cancer may first be discovered after finding a lump in the armpit (axilla) or a cancer lump (secondary) in another organ such as in lungs (seen in a chest X-ray) or the liver or bone.

Investigations

Screening tests for breast cancer were discussed in Section 2. In an examination for possible breast cancer the doctor will first look for a breast lump. The doctor will take note of the relative hardness of any lump and an irregular outline or attachment to the skin, muscle or other tissue. The doctor will examine lymph nodes in the axilla (armpit) or elsewhere for evidence of enlargement and may also examine the chest and abdomen for possible evidence of lumps or spread into other organs such as the lungs, liver, bone, ovaries, etc.

A number of investigations are available for detecting breast cancer. Breast X-rays (mammograms) may show the type of lump and the general condition of the breast. Ultrasound and CT scans may also be helpful, although as a rule they give little further information.

The most important investigation is a biopsy. In many cases a needle biopsy may be carried out on an outpatient basis. Sometimes it is better for a surgeon to take a larger biopsy in an operating theatre: this is the most reliable method of diagnosis. If a surgical biopsy is carried out with the frozen-section pathology technique (described in Section 2), the surgeon may be able to go ahead with any necessary surgical operation without further delay.

If, after a doctor's examination, a breast lump is thought to be cancer, and especially if it is an advanced cancer, other general investigations will be arranged. These may include chest X-rays, liver ultrasound scans, bone scans or CT scans, which may provide evidence of possible spread to lungs, liver or bone. The involvement of any of these organs should be known before any major surgery is carried out on the breast. If other organs are affected, some form of treatment other than breast surgery may be more appropriate.

Treatment

Treatment of breast cancer will depend on whether the cancer was detected early and is likely to be cured by surgery or other local treatment, or whether it is so advanced that cure by surgical treatment of the breast alone is not possible.

Prevention

There is no simple specific way of preventing development of breast cancer apart from possibly a change in Western diets and the lifestyles of girls and young women in high-risk communities. However, studies are being conducted on the use of the anti-oestrogen hormone compound tamoxifen, given over a period of up to five years (or even longer in special circumstances), to prevent breast cancer developing in women who are at special risk. These include those with a high incidence of breast cancer in their immediate family or those who have already had cancer in one breast. The results of these trials, especially in deciding who would most likely benefit, are at this time inconclusive. Whether there would be any advantage in using the newer anti-oestrogens Femara or Armidex has yet to be fully tested.

Women in Asian countries have a lower incidence of breast cancer and premenstrual syndrome than women in Western societies. Asian women have a diet high in soybeans and other foods that contain the natural plant hormone substances known as phytoestrogens. There are ongoing studies designed to determine whether the phytoestrogens from these dietary products reduce the risk of breast diseases, including cancer.

A major advance has been the recognition that in certain families specific gene mutations predispose to breast cancer. There are now special DNA or gene tests for these mutations to determine individuals at risk. Such women may then have intensive surveillance.

Early breast cancer
Surgery and/or radiotherapy

The treatment of early breast cancer has, for many years, been an emotive topic.

Previously, surgeons considered that the best chance of curing breast cancer was the total removal of the breast and all of the draining lymph nodes in the armpit. This operation, known as a radical mastectomy, was performed for many years and cured many women of breast cancer. However, it was greatly feared because of the mutilation involved, as well as the risk of lymphoedoma (arm swelling). Over the last 20 years large clinical trials in the USA, Europe and Australia involving thousands of women have, thankfully, dramatically improved the situation. Firstly these randomised clinical studies have shown that, in women with relatively small tumours, it is possible to simply remove that part of the breast containing the cancer. This is called a segmental or partial mastectomy or sometimes a 'lumpectomy'. It is usually followed by radiotherapy to the affected breast in case any cancer cells have escaped the surgery and remain somewhere in the breast. Similarly trials, still underway, suggest it is only necessary to remove the so-called sentinel lymph node (or sometimes two or three nodes) in the armpit. This can be identified by injecting a coloured dye into the skin of the breast near the cancer. Alternatively a radio-isotope tracer may be used. This is similar to the procedure used in surgery for melanoma. Removed nodes are then examined by the pathologist for cancer cells. The results of this are critical in determining the patient's outlook. Generally if a sentinel lymph node is involved then some form of additional therapy is given (see below). The removal of only one or two nodes from the armpit reduces the risk of lymphoedema developing in the arm. (There are up to about 30 nodes in total in each armpit, but the sentinel node or nodes are most likely to be first to be involved with any cancer spread.)

It is important that the patient receive a careful explanation of the various treatment alternatives available. Obviously the patient's wishes should be taken into consideration. If the patient would prefer to have the breast with a cancer in it totally removed, then this treatment can be offered. On the other hand, where a patient has a wish for less radical surgery with breast conservation this is now usually very appropriate. Results are essentially the same.

Adjuvant chemotherapy

It has long been recognised that many women, particularly those with lymph-node involvement, have an undetectable spread of some cancer cells to other parts of the body, such as the lungs, liver, bones or elsewhere (micrometastases). These are the cause of subsequent relapse or recurrence of the disease months or years after apparently successful surgery. If chemotherapy or hormonal therapy is given soon after surgery, these small but undetected clumps of scattered cancer cells, if present, are more likely to be destroyed than if they are allowed to grow and actually cause symptoms or signs. In women who have had an early breast cancer removed that involved lymph nodes in the axilla, a program of chemotherapy and/or hormone therapy is usually given after the surgery. This is known as adjuvant therapy, the chemotherapy being an adjunct or assistant to the surgery. Women given adjuvant therapy are less likely to develop secondary cancer and are therefore more likely to be cured. As indicated in Section 2, the chemotherapy must be given skilfully and the effects watched closely, as side effects are common. The specific types of therapy will depend on a number of factors including the woman's age, the size of the primary cancer and whether hormone receptors are present in the cancer specimen. Adjuvant chemotherapy is more appropriate for younger women, who appear to benefit more and also better tolerate the effects of chemotherapy than older women. Hormone therapy is usually more appropriate for older women. For many years tamoxifen, which antagonises oestrogen, had been used. It is now being replaced by the drug Arimidex, which prevents synthesis of oestrogen (see 'Hormone therapy' in Section 2).

About 20% of women will have increased amounts of a

cancer-cell surface receptor, a protein called HER2. They may be treated with an artificially manufactured antibody called Herceptin. In many treatment centres women will be asked to participate in clinical trials of new treatments being studied. These trials are quite safe and offer patients the chance to receive some of the newer therapies. Patients entering such trials are carefully monitored and are contributing to knowledge that may help other women in the future.

Locally advanced breast cancer

Rarely women may present with a breast cancer that has become locally advanced. Such cancers are large and may ulcerate (fungate) through the skin of the breast or the nipple, or may possibly be fixed to the chest wall. Commonly such women will have enlarged axillary lymph nodes. Unfortunately the outlook for such women is much poorer than those with early or smaller cancers. However, a small percentage can be cured, and many will gain some years of good-quality life.

A small biopsy of the tumour is taken to confirm the diagnosis and is also sent to the pathologist for assessment of its hormone-receptor status (oestrogen- and progestrogen-receptor status) as well as the HER2 receptor. Depending on the age of the women, these patients may be treated with vigorous chemotherapy to shrink the cancer mass. This is often enough to then allow surgery in which usually the cancer and the entire breast is removed. This is then generally followed by radiation therapy to the site of surgery. In some rare cases, if the local cancer is very big or fungating through the skin, the chemotherapy may be more concentrated in the cancer if given directly into an artery, or arteries, supplying the breast with blood. This will give an even greater chance of shrinking the cancer sufficiently to allow its removal by surgery (see Section 2).

Older women, particularly if their cancer is oestrogen-receptor positive, may be simply treated initially with tamoxifen or Arimidex, which will usually lead to slow shrinkage of the cancer lump. This may eventually result in a much smaller tumour that can be surgically removed and followed by radiation therapy to the breast.

Patients so treated may remain well for some years. Often for very elderly patients that is all that is required as they may have other coexisting diseases (e.g. heart or cerebro-vascular disease). For younger women a small percentage may be cured, but often, unfortunately, the disease may either relapse locally or, because of distant spread, metastases may appear.

Metastatic breast cancer

In this situation, possibly many months or years after treatment of the initial primary breast cancer, spread of the disease may become apparent by the appearance of metastases. Bone metastases are one of the more common forms of presentation, and women may present with non-specific symptoms such as backache, or even what is called a pathological fracture of a bone, where trivial trauma leads to a bone fracture. X-rays generally demonstrate changes in the bone where they have become thinned by the presence of the cancer. Various scans are then done to assess the spread of the cancer.

Similarly, metastases in the liver or lung may be discovered. Rarely, but generally in the late stages of the disease, it is possible to develop metastases in the brain. Again, treatment, although not curative, may allow women many months or even several years of good-quality life. The best outcomes occur when the original tumour or metastatic tumour is shown to contain hormone receptors. Treatment may then just consist of hormonal therapy such as the drugs tamoxifen or Arimidex.

Locally troublesome symptoms (e.g. bone pain) can often also be dealt with by radiotherapy. Bone fractures are attended to by the orthopaedic surgeons with pinning and plating as necessary followed by radiation therapy.

Women with cancers that do not contain hormone receptors usually require a course of chemotherapy. Various combinations of the anti-cancer drugs (described in Section 2) may be used, and this may be combined with the monoclonal antibody Herceptin, if the cancer is positive for the HER2 receptor.

It is important that complications are also adequately treated, to relieve symptoms such as those caused by accumulation of fluid in the pleural cavity or abdominal cavity and provide appropriate treatment of pain.

Some years ago very high-dose chemotherapy with bone-marrow transplantation was trialled in advanced breast cancer.

However, it appears that this therapy, which is very toxic, is no better than standard chemotherapy.

Many thousands of women are entering various clinical trials of newer drugs that are being continuously developed. In this way over the last few decades the outlook for women with breast cancer has been dramatically improved, with a significant reduction in deaths.

Breast prosthesis and reconstruction

Fortunately many women can now avoid mastectomy and loss of the breast. However, for those who require mastectomy this can be emotionally traumatic. After the loss of a breast, many women feel quite depressed, even humiliated, and require sympathetic help and understanding.

Prosthetic breast padding has improved, and types are now available that allow normal activity, even swimming, without detection. In other cases plastic or reconstructive breast surgery may be considered. These procedures are usually not advised until at least a couple of years after mastectomy, in order to be as sure as possible that recurrence of the cancer is unlikely. On the other hand, some specialised plastic surgeons are now offering reconstructive surgery to replace the breast immediately after its removal. Such procedures offer considerable emotional benefit to some women.

Emotional support and the understanding of family and friends are essential for most women who have had breast cancer, even if they have not had a mastectomy. As breast cancer is one of the most common cancers in Western societies, many cities have mastectomy support groups that women are welcome to join, and company and advice from group members can be of great help. Local state cancer councils can advise on the contact details of such support groups.

CANCERS OF THE DIGESTIVE SYSTEM

Cancer of the oesophagus

The oesophagus is the hollow food passage that passes from the mouth and pharynx through the chest to the stomach (in the abdomen). Cancer of the oesophagus is a common disease in Asian and some African countries, as well as Russia and Scandinavia, but is less common in people of Anglo-Celtic origin. The reason for this difference in incidence is not fully understood, but diet plays a significant role. Northern China has a very high incidence, caused by a fungus that grows on poorly stored food. Cancer of the oesophagus is more common in men, particularly those who smoke and drink alcohol to excess. Oesophageal cancers in men are usually in the middle or lower oesophagus. Cancers in the upper oesophagus are more common in women.

There are two types of oesophageal cancer. The commonest is squamous cancer in the upper or middle oesophagus, and the other is adenocarcinoma, which occurs in the lower oesophagus close to the junction with the stomach.

Symptoms and signs

Unfortunately, cancer of the oesophagus is often relatively advanced at the time of diagnosis. The most common symptom is difficulty with swallowing. This is first noted when swallowing solids, which seem to get caught in the throat or chest. Later there is difficulty in swallowing liquids. A person with cancer of the oesophagus will soon lose weight, become quite wasted and even dehydrated.

Investigations

Barium-swallow or barium-meal X-rays (see Section 2) will usually show an obstructive or irregular narrowing at the site of the cancer.

Oesophagoscopy is carried out and the doctor can usually see an irregular or ulcerated cancer. A biopsy is taken to establish the diagnosis by microscopic examination.

Unfortunately, cancers of the oesophagus will have often spread up and down the mucous membrane (lining) of the oeso-phagus and into lymph nodes and other structures in the chest before the patient notices many symptoms. Thus, by the time the patient has consulted a doctor the cancers generally have a relatively low cure rate.

Treatment

The best hope of cure is by surgery. The oesophagus is removed and either the stomach or a section of bowel is used as a replacement for the passage of food.

In some cancer-treatment clinics chemotherapy or combined chemo/radiotherapy is used prior to attempts at curative surgery. Studies are being made in a number of world centres to determine which combinations of chemotherapy and radiotherapy and surgery achieve best results. Although the outlook for people with oesophageal cancer must still be circumspect, more encouraging results are being reported from some centres.

Sometimes it is not possible to attempt to remove the cancer, and the most helpful treatment is for the surgeon to pass a plastic tube (stent) through the oesophagus into the stomach to allow the patient to swallow food. Otherwise, some alternative food passage (such as a transplanted section of bowel) or another method of feeding may be required. Radiotherapy, sometimes combined with chemotherapy, may be used in this palliative way. This can result in cancer shrinkage, often relieving symptoms for a time.

Cancer of the stomach

Cancer of the stomach was once one of the most common cancers in the Western world but is no longer so. Stomach cancer is uncommon before the age of 40 years but increases in incidence with age, reaching a peak between the ages of 60 and 65. Males are affected about two or three times more commonly than females.

Cancer of the stomach has a distinct racial or geographic association. It is about seven times more common in Japan and Korea and three or four times more common in Eastern Europe than it is in Australia or the USA. Epidemiological studies suggest that it has a direct relationship to diet. People who have a diet high in animal fats and low in fresh fruit and vegetables are at greater risk of stomach cancer. It may also be related to a high intake of chemical food preservatives and food subject to other methods of preservation and preparation, such as the smoking of fish or meat. The high intake of smoked fish in Japan has been incriminated; there is also a high incidence of this cancer among the people of northern Iceland, who eat large amounts of crude smoked salmon, whereas there is a lower incidence in the people of southern Iceland, who have a different diet. In Korea the custom of eating a great deal of red pepper and possibly other spices in food is thought to be significant in increasing the risk.

The decreasing incidence of stomach cancer in modern industrialised societies appears to be the result of the greater availability of fresh fruit and vegetables due to improved transport and the use of refrigeration rather than chemical preservatives, additives or smoking.

There are also a number of rare conditions that result in a higher risk of stomach cancer: pernicious anaemia, chronic gastritis, polyps in the stomach and possibly gastric ulcers. Tobacco smokers also have an increased risk compared to non-smokers.

Symptoms and signs

Like cancer of the oesophagus, stomach cancer is often quite advanced before pain or other symptoms are noticed. The earliest symptom is usually some vague indigestion that gradually becomes worse. Persistent indigestion occurring for the first time in someone over the age of 40 years must always be considered with suspicion.

Sometimes an early feature is loss of appetite, especially for certain foods, particularly meat. Other symptoms may be a feeling of being full or even feeling 'blown up' in the stomach after eating small amounts of food, or vomiting after food, particularly if vomiting becomes frequent or regular. This may indicate blockage of the outlet of the stomach. Pain is sometimes the first symptom, but, as mentioned, when pain is persistent, the cancer is often quite advanced. Some patients may actually vomit fresh blood (haematemesis).

Sometimes a patient may not be aware of any symptoms but has found a lump in the upper abdomen. In others complaints of weakness and tiredness due to anaemia or recent unexplained weight loss may have caused the patient to seek medical attention. Occasionally the first evidence of illness is caused by the cancer spreading to other organs, presenting an enlarged liver or jaundice. Pain in the back can be caused by the cancer spreading to the pancreas or into lymph nodes behind the stomach.

The doctor will look for a swelling or lump in the abdomen, evidence of an enlarged liver or lymph nodes (especially an enlarged lymph node in the left side of the neck), evidence of spread into the pelvis or an ovary (felt on vaginal or rectal examination), and evidence of fluid in the abdominal cavity. There might also be weight loss or anaemia (due to the cancer bleeding into the stomach cavity).

Investigations

The doctor may test for blood in the faeces or test the blood for iron-deficiency anaemia or other abnormalities.

Gastroscopy (see Section 2) is now commonly performed as a first investigation. Through a gastroscope a cancer may be seen as an ulcer with raised edges, a mass or a rigid abnormal distortion of the stomach wall. A biopsy can also be taken to confirm the diagnosis. This is necessary to distinguish gastric cancer from other cancer types, such as gastric lymphoma.

Barium-meal X-ray films and screening may show an ulcer (usually with raised, rounded edges) or a lump on the stomach wall looking something like a small cauliflower. The X-rays and screening may alternatively show a blocked stomach, a change in the stomach's shape or size (bigger or shrunken and smaller), or a more rigid and stiff-walled stomach. However, X-rays will not show all cancers in the stomach, and other tests are also needed. However, since gastroscopic examinations have become reliable and easily performed, these radiological investigations are now done less commonly.

CT scans may be useful to determine the size, extent and spread of a gastric cancer (e.g. spread into the pancreas behind the stomach, into adjacent lymph nodes or into the liver).

Treatment

The only potentially curative treatment for cancer of the stomach is surgery in which the stomach is completely removed (total gastrectomy), mostly removed (sub-total gastrectomy) or partly removed (partial gastrectomy).

If a cancer has already spread beyond the stomach, cure may not be possible, but it may still be possible to give the patient relief of symptoms by a bypass operation to relieve blockage.

After total gastrectomy the small intestine is joined to the oesophagus or, in the case of a sub-total or partial gastrectomy, the small intestine is joined to the remaining part of the stomach to allow food to pass through normally. With no stomach present or only a small part of the stomach present, the patient can eat only small meals and therefore needs to eat frequently to avoid excessive weight loss. Without a stomach the patient may also develop a form of pernicious anaemia. This can be prevented by injections of vitamin B12.

The results of surgery alone in treating stomach cancer have been disappointing in the past. In general the smaller a cancer is at surgery the better the results. For this reason, gastroscopy and other diagnostic tests may be used to look for evidence of cancer as soon as a patient complains to a doctor of early symptoms, especially if the patient is a male over the age of 40 years. In some countries, and especially in Japan where stomach cancer is common, screening tests are often carried out for people at risk even if they do not have any symptoms. If stomach cancers are found while they are small and in the early stages (as is now often the case in Japan), the results of treatment by operation are good, with a high rate of cure. However, this is not often the case in Western societies, where stomach cancer is less common and is not often diagnosed until troublesome symptoms have developed, by which time the cancers are advanced and unlikely to be cured by surgery alone.

Anti-cancer drugs do not cure this cancer, but they may be useful in treating people whose cancers cannot be cured by operation. The drugs will often make the cancers smaller and may give the patients good relief, possibly for several months.

More recently, anti-cancer drugs have been given to some patients before the operation (induction or neoadjuvant chemotherapy, see Section 2). There is some evidence that if the cancers are made smaller by the drugs before a gastrectomy is carried out, the results and the chances of cure will be better. Often chemotherapy may be given after surgery if the lymph nodes are involved, and this has been shown to improve chances of survival.

In some cancer centres studies are under way to determine whether giving the drugs pre-operatively by direct infusion into the artery that supplies blood to the stomach results in more effective reduction of the cancer before surgery.

Cancer of the liver

Primary liver cancer (hepatoma)

Cancer starting in liver cells (primary cancer) is uncommon in ethnic Europeans but is a major problem in Africans, South East Asians, Chinese and Japanese. It represents some 50% of all cancers in African Bantu men. These differences appear to reflect hygiene, diet and food-storage practices. Chronic liver infection due to hepatitis B and hepatitis C is responsible for much of the increased incidence in Asia. Certain fungi-producing toxins (aflatoxins) and contaminated food in parts of Africa also play a major role.

Primary liver cancer also sometimes develops in people with longstanding cirrhosis (a fibrotic degeneration) of the liver, as a result of excessive alcohol consumption or other causes, and this is the most common cause in Western countries.

Symptoms and signs

The first evidence of primary liver cancer may be general ill health (loss of appetite, weight loss, weakness and debility) or liver enlargement with pain in the upper abdomen, swelling, jaundice or fluid in the abdominal cavity (ascites).

Investigations

Investigations that may help include CT scans, ultrasounds, sometimes arteriography and especially liver biopsy. Blood tests for liver function, for anaemia and for blood-chemical changes are often helpful too. A special blood-tumour marker test called alpha-feto-protein estimation usually gives an elevated reading in people with this cancer; it usually falls to normal levels if the cancer has been cured. Progressive alpha-feto-protein tests may thus give useful evidence of the effectiveness of treatment.

Treatment

The treatment of hepatoma is only successful if the disease is detected when it is confined to a part of the liver that can be removed by surgical operation. Unfortunately, as the cancer has usually spread widely in the liver when first detected, cure is usually not possible. It is possible, however, to prolong life, sometimes for many months, by injecting cancer masses in the liver with cold alcohol, microwave needle probes or with freezing probes (cryosurgery). In some patients a catheter can be placed in the main artery to the liver and injected with either chemotherapy or radioactive micro-beads. This can cause shrinkage of the cancer and relief of symptoms, and occasionally, but very rarely, the cancer can then be resected.

Secondary (metastatic) liver cancer

Although primary liver cancer is uncommon in people of European races, the liver is one of the most common sites of secondary cancer in all races, including Europeans. Cancers of the digestive tract, especially the stomach, pancreas, colon and rectum, commonly spread via the bloodstream to the liver. Cancers of almost any other tissue may also spread to the liver, but breast cancer, lung cancer and melanoma are especially likely to do this.

Secondary cancers in the liver cause it to enlarge. It may become uncomfortable or even painful; jaundice often develops and fluid may accumulate in the abdominal cavity. A person with secondary liver cancer sooner or later notices loss of appetite, loss of weight and loss of energy. Breathlessness may also be a symptom.

Investigations

The doctor will look for the features mentioned above and may arrange investigations to help establish the diagnosis. The most helpful investigations are usually a CT scan, ultrasound and sometimes arteriography. A liver biopsy, either carried out with a special needle through the lower chest or abdominal wall under local anaesthesia or done during an operation, may be required to be sure of the diagnosis. This biopsy is not always needed if a primary cancer has been previously recognised, however.

If the site of a primary cancer that has spread to the liver is not known, investigations may sometimes be carried out to discover where the secondary cancer in the liver originated. Various blood tests can help in this situation.

Treatment

Secondary cancer in the liver is usually not curable. A potential for cure exists if there are a small number of secondaries in one part of the liver that can be surgically excised. However, this is not common. In most people the secondary cancers are spread throughout most parts of the liver.

For patients with liver metastases that cannot be surgically excised many approaches to treatment have been used. If the primary cancer is known to be sensitive to chemotherapy (e.g. breast cancer, lymphoma, testicular cancer, colorectal cancer), then the various drug combinations that are known to be effective in these diseases can be used. Alternative therapies have included direct intra-arterial infusion of cytotoxic drugs via a small catheter placed in the hepatic artery, which supplies blood to the liver. This can be connected to a small pump that can be placed under the skin in the anterior abdominal wall. It is possible for these pumps to infuse medication over many months. In some patients this can lead to significant shrinkage of the cancers and improvement in quality of life.

It is also possible to carry out what is called chemo-embolisation, in which micro-beads are combined with chemotherapy and injected via catheter into the hepatic artery. Similarly, radioactive micro-beads can also be injected via the catheter.

Other alternatives are radio-frequency ablation via micro-wave probes directly inserted into liver metastases, alcohol injections into the metastases and injection of the metastases with a freezing probe. This freezing probe causes the secondary cancer deposits to be frozen, and the cells are killed when the freezing thaws.

An approach being studied in some highly specialised surgical oncology centres is for the surgeon to isolate the liver from the general body circulation and infuse very high doses of chemotherapy into the liver circulation for an hour or so. From early studies some temporary success has been reported using this treatment, but no long-term cures are apparent as yet.

For most patients the disease will subsequently progress and ultimately prove fatal. However, with some simple measures it is possible to make the last weeks and days of such patients really quite comfortable. Corticosteroid drugs are very effective at relieving the pain and tenderness associated with the liver-capsule distension, and various morphine derivatives will also relieve pain and give a sense of wellbeing.

Cancer of the gall bladder and bile ducts

These are relatively uncommon cancers in Western countries although quite common in parts of some countries, such as southern India. Cancer of the gall bladder is usually associated with gallstones (cholelithiasis) that have been present for many years, particularly in older women. By contrast bile-duct cancer is slightly more common in men.

The removal of gall bladders with gallstones, especially in young women, is often recommended to reduce the risk of subsequent cancer.

Early cancer may occasionally be found unexpectedly on pathological examination of the gall bladder after it has been removed for chronic inflammation or gallstones. In such cases cure of the cancer may have been achieved simply by the removal of the gall bladder.

If it is not diagnosed early, cancer of the gall bladder may cause persistent pain in the upper right side of the abdomen, with evidence of inflammation of the gall bladder, or it may cause a swelling or lump felt in the upper abdomen under the ribs on the right side.

The first indication of cancer of the gall bladder, and more especially cancer of the bile ducts, may be jaundice due to the blockage of the flow of bile from the liver. The jaundice is often accompanied by a severe itch of the patient's skin.

Cancer of the gall bladder tends to spread into the liver as well as into nearby lymph nodes. Once this has happened, it is virtually incurable by surgery and does not respond well to radiotherapy. It also has a reputation for not responding well to chemotherapy, although good response to intra-arterial chemotherapy (see Section 2) and cure with following surgery has been reported. In advanced cases jaundice and itch, if present, can usually be relieved by an operation in which the obstruction to bile flow is bypassed, allowing the bile to flow into the small intestine by another route.

Cancer of the pancreas

Cancer of the pancreas has become increasingly common in Westernised societies over recent years. It is now the fourth most common cause of cancer death in males in Australia and the third most common cause of cancer death in males in the US. Although it is slightly more common in men, its incidence is similar in both men and women. Risk factors for its development include smoking, diabetes, chronic pancreatitis, obesity and a high-fat diet.

Symptoms and signs

Cancer of the pancreas often invades or compresses the bile duct draining from the liver, as it passes through the pancreas. As the cancer grows, it commonly blocks the bile duct, obstructing the flow of bile from the liver into the intestine and resulting in jaundice. The level of jaundice may be quite intense. The jaundice is sometimes painless, although there is often pain felt deep in the upper abdomen and passing through to the back.

As the jaundice develops, the patient's skin may become very itchy. The liver and gall bladder often become enlarged due to obstruction of the bile duct. Occasionally the cancer can be felt as a lump in the upper abdomen.

Weight loss may be the first feature of this disease. Anorexia (loss of appetite) is usual, and diarrhoea may also be present.

Investigations

As the pancreas lies across the back of the upper abdomen behind the stomach and other organs, it has been difficult in the past to examine or investigate. However, in recent years improved methods of investigating and imaging the pancreas have become available.

Ultrasound, CT and MRI scans have been of some help in detecting cancers, although early detection of the smaller and potentially curable cancers before they cause symptoms is rare.

Examination of the pancreatic duct using an endoscope passed orally and through the stomach into the duodenum (ERCP examination) has allowed pancreatic secretions to be examined for cancer cells and X-rays to be taken of the duct. These may be helpful in detecting evidence of some pancreatic cancers at an early stage.

PET scanning using a glucose product (fluorodeoxyglucose) as a tracer appears to be highly successful in identifying pancreatic cancer localisation (see Section 2). The serum marker CA19.9 is also helpful in diagnosis and in management.

Needle biopsy of any lump in the pancreas under CT guidance

is the most useful method of establishing a diagnosis, although this procedure does have risks and is not always reliable.

Treatment

At the time of detection cancer of the pancreas has often spread to the liver as well as to lymph nodes and cure by surgery is no longer possible. However, some small cancers can be resected in a major surgical operation with some prospect of cure. In some cancer-treatment clinics a combination of chemotherapy with radiotherapy is used prior to surgery to improve the chance of complete surgical removal (induction or neoadjuvant therapy). Alternatively, this treatment may be given after surgery. In some highly specialised surgical oncology centres some success has also been reported with chemotherapy given by intra-arterial infusion before surgery.

For those suffering jaundice due to pancreatic cancer obstructing the bile duct, relief can usually be achieved by a surgical operation in which the obstruction to the bile duct is bypassed.

Cancer of the small intestine

Cancer of the small intestine is rare. The most common of the rare primary malignant tumours of the small intestine are a lymphoma and a tumour called a carcinoid (cancer-like) tumour. These are rare causes of abdominal pain, bowel bleeding and small bowel obstruction. They are usually treated by a surgical operation in which the tumour is removed along with part of the bowel.

Carcinoid tumours may occur anywhere in the alimentary (digestive) tract. That is, they may occur anywhere between the mouth and the anus. However, the most common site of a carcinoid tumour is the appendix. Most carcinoids in the appendix (and in fact most small carcinoids) are not malignant. Sometimes when an appendix has been removed, a small carcinoid tumour may be found in it. In most such cases the tumour has been cured by removal of the appendix and further treatment is not necessary.

When a carcinoid tumour is found in the small intestine, it is more likely to be larger, more likely to be malignant and may have already spread to the liver. Secondary carcinoids in the liver may release certain biochemical substances that can cause bouts of diarrhoea, flushing of the skin of the face or wheezing of the lungs. Treatment can be given to control these episodes, but once this tumour has spread into the liver a complete cure is unlikely.

A rare tumour originating in connective tissue is the so-called gastrointestinal stromal tumour or GIST. This tumour has an unusual protein (called a mutated signal receptor) on its cell surfaces and responds dramatically to a new 'targeted' drug called Glivec. The drug specifically inhibits the abnormal receptor, blocking transmission of growth signals in the tumour cells, thus stopping cancer-cell division. This drug is given orally. It is also extremely effective in treating chronic myeloid leukaemia.

Cancer of the large bowel

In Western societies the large bowel is the most common site of primary cancer other than skin cancer. In the adult populations (both male and female) of Australia and New Zealand bowel cancer is responsible for more deaths than any other cancer. In the adult population of the USA lung cancer causes more deaths but bowel cancer is next.

Bowel cancer is occasionally seen in young adults and even in children but is not commonly seen until after the age of 40 years. Thereafter the incidence rises with age, reaching a peak between 60 and 75.

As discussed in Section 1, cancer of the large bowel is most common in societies where the food intake is relatively high in meat and animal fats and relatively low in fibre. Fibre is a greater component of wholemeal grains, fruit and vegetables.

Polyps in the large bowel also predispose people to cancer and, if present, should be removed to avoid the risk of malignant change. People who have had polyps removed should be kept under regular colonoscopy observation in case more develop.

The uncommon hereditary condition familial adenomatous polyposis is one in which about half of the members of an affected family are likely to develop multiple polyps. It is a highly pre-malignant condition, and all close blood relatives in an affected family should be kept under regular observation. If polyps are found, the large bowel should be removed to prevent the development of cancer later in life. If this is not done, most people will have developed a bowel cancer by the age of about 40 years.

Other conditions associated with an increased risk of large-bowel cancer are the inflammatory bowel diseases ulcerative colitis and, to a lesser extent, granular (Crohn's) colitis. People with longstanding and extensive ulcerative colitis must be kept under close and regular observation and in some circumstances may be well advised to have the colon removed as a precautionary measure.

Close relatives of any patient with large-bowel cancer have a slightly increased risk of developing a similar cancer. This is termed hereditary non-polyposis colorectal cancer, reflecting a specific gene mutation. There are also rarer genetic syndromes leading to colorectal cancer.

After successful treatment of one large-bowel cancer, the patient has a rather greater than average risk of developing a second cancer in the large bowel, although by far the majority of such patients never develop a new cancer. However, regular follow-up observation is desirable for all patients after treatment for bowel cancer, as for all patients treated for other types of cancer. It is standard practice for patients to have a follow-up colonoscopy within the first 12 months following surgery for colorectal cancer. This is to ensure that a second cancer or polyps are not missed.

Symptoms and signs

The most common symptoms associated with large-bowel cancer are a change in bowel habits (constipation or diarrhoea or alternating constipation and diarrhoea), rectal bleeding or a feeling of incomplete evacuation of the rectum after going to the toilet. Some patients may not notice any symptoms until the cancer has caused bowel obstruction. This may cause abdominal colic, constipation and abdominal distension.

Other features of large-bowel cancer may be debility, weight loss, tiredness and lassitude (sometimes due to anaemia) or features of liver enlargement with jaundice due to liver metastases.

The doctor may be able to feel a lump or localised swelling in the abdomen or, on examination through the anus, a mass in the rectum. There may be evidence of blood in the faeces. In the case of obstructive bowel cancer, evidence of bowel obstruction with abdominal distension or swelling may be found.

Investigations

Investigations that may help in establishing a diagnosis include examination with a flexible sigmoidoscope through the anus. About 50% of large-bowel cancers are in the rectum or the lowest part of the colon just above the rectum, and most of these can be seen and biopsied through the sigmoidoscope. This can be done as an outpatient procedure (see Section 2).

Examination with a fibre-optic colonoscope, however, requires sedation or possibly an anaesthetic, but this examination will allow the whole length of the large bowel to be examined visually and for biopsies to be taken from any part of the length of the colon. These are performed in day-care outpatient centres. Less commonly, barium enemas are done to visualise the colon and rectum.

Blood studies are carried out for evidence of anaemia and changes in biochemistry of the blood or impaired liver function. One particular blood test useful for the diagnosis, management and study of a patient with large-bowel cancer is the carcinoembryonic antigen (CEA) test. This test is usually strongly positive in people with large-bowel cancer and becomes negative after successful treatment. If it becomes positive again after treatment, it may suggest recurrence of the cancer.

CT scans may also be done to look for any evidence of secondary liver cancer.

Treatment

Large-bowel cancer requires surgery to remove that part of the bowel containing the cancer together with draining lymph nodes into which the cancer may have spread. Generally the bowel is joined together again (anastomosed) and the patient can return to normal life.

When the cancer is very low in the rectum, it may be necessary to remove the anus as well as the rectum; in this case an opening (colostomy) for the lower bowel is made in the abdominal wall to allow evacuation of faeces. The patient wears a bag over the colostomy, and the bowel empties at regular intervals into the bag. The patient learns to empty the bag at convenient times and recovers to live an active and virtually normal life.

Colostomy associations or groups have branches in many large cities. These groups offer support and advice on learning to live with a colostomy and the other social adjustments that may worry patients.

In the hands of specialist colorectal surgeons, and depending on the stage of the tumour, some 50–75% of patients will be cured. With or without a colostomy most of these then return to normal life.

If a cancer first appears with a bowel obstruction, it may be necessary to perform a temporary colostomy to relieve the obstruction. Usually the cancer is removed at a further surgical operation three or four weeks later, and the colostomy is closed, resulting in a return to a normal passage of bowel actions.

The outcome for patients with colorectal cancers has improved significantly in recent years. An advance in rectal cancer has been, for some patients, treatment prior to surgery with a combination of chemotherapy and radiotherapy. This has reduced the need for a colostomy as well as reducing the risk of local recurrence of the cancer in the pelvis. A second major advance has come from clinical trials using some of the newer anti-cancer drugs after surgery in patients who are found to have lymph-node involvement. These have reduced the chance of metastatic disease spread or recurrence. This is a form of adjuvant chemotherapy (see Section 2).

Follow-up care

As for all patients who have had treatment for cancer, regular follow-up consultations and care are required for patients who have had a bowel cancer removed. A follow-up colonoscopy is usually done within a year of the operation. There is always a risk of secondary cancer showing up in the liver or elsewhere, and there may be a risk of another cancer developing, which can be effectively treated if detected while still small. In the case of bowel cancer, any secondary cancer usually shows up within two years; it is uncommon for it to appear after five years. If the patient has been followed up for five years without evidence of recurrence, he or she is usually considered to be cured.

If the cancer has spread to the liver, cure is rarely possible except, for example, in occasional cases where there is a small number of metastases that can be surgically resected.

Secondary spread to the liver can sometimes be controlled for up to two to three years with the newer types of chemotherapy. The recent development of an implantable pump to continuously infuse cytotoxic drugs into the artery supplying blood to the liver has shown encouraging results as far as improving the patient's quality of life and life expectancy are concerned but is very rarely curative.

Cancer of the anus

Cancer of the anus is not common but may present as a lump, an ulcer, bleeding or pain in the anal region. Sometimes it may develop in a pre-existing benign lesion such as a papilloma (a fern-like growth from the bowel lining), a patch of leukoplakia (white patch) or in a longstanding anal fissure (a split in the wall of the opening of the anus).

Most cancers of the anus are similar in type to SCC of skin but behave more aggressively in that they tend to spread to lymph nodes in the groin or pelvis at an earlier stage and often require radical treatment to achieve the best chances of cure.

Treatment

A biopsy is taken to confirm the exact diagnosis. Treatment is generally a combination of chemotherapy and radiotherapy over several weeks as an outpatient. This approach has a high cure rate. This means extensive surgery and a colostomy can be avoided in many patients unless they present with very advanced disease or have not completely responded to the course of chemotherapy and radiotherapy.

CANCERS OF THE HEAD AND NECK

Cancers of the lips, mouth, tongue, nasal cavity, the paranasal air sinuses, throat, larynx and pharynx (the passage at the back of the nose and mouth) constitute about 5% of all cancers encountered in Western countries. Most of these cancers are similar pathologically to SCCs of the skin but tend to behave in a more malignant and aggressive fashion. As a rule, the further away the cancers are from the lips the more aggressively they behave.

Smoking is the major cause of this group of cancers. It has been estimated that cancers in the mouth and throat are about six times more common in smokers, and this is increased to about 15 times if the smokers are also heavy consumers of alcohol. Other pre-malignant conditions that predispose to cancer in the mouth include leukoplakia, papillomata and chronic irritation from such causes as ill-fitting dentures or jagged teeth (see Section 1). Cancer of the buccal mucosa (cheek lining) is common in India and South East Asia, where betel-nut chewing is a common practice. It is especially common in people who mix betel-nut with tobacco leaf or lime and hold the mixture in the cheek pouch.

Cancers of the lips

Because of their high visibility cancers of the lips are usually diagnosed at an early, potentially curable, stage. They may develop as a thickening in an area of hyperkeratosis (sun damage), more often on the lower lip. They tend to ulcerate, possibly bleed, or may form a lump. They may later spread to lymph nodes under the jaw and in the neck, where they may form palpable lumps.

A biopsy is taken to confirm the diagnosis, and thereafter treatment is usually by surgical excision, with good results both cosmetically (in appearance) and in eventual cure rates. Radiotherapy may also be used with good results.

For larger cancers of the lips, either radical surgery removing a large part of the lip (with some form of plastic or reconstructive surgery to fashion a new lip) or radiotherapy may be used, and the chances of cure are still quite good.

If hard enlarged lymph nodes are present either when the patient is first seen or at a later follow-up visit to the doctor, then these are best treated by a surgical excision known as a block dissection (an operation to remove all lymph nodes in one block of tissue).

Occasionally a patient first consults a doctor when the cancer is very large and ulcerating and possibly the whole of the lip is involved with cancer. In these patients considerable success can be achieved with induction chemotherapy prior to surgery or radio-therapy. If the expertise is available, pre-operative chemotherapy given by intra-arterial infusion is even more effective in reducing very advanced cancers to smaller cancers that will be more curable by surgery or radiotherapy, or if necessary both (see Section 2).

Cancers of the floor of the mouth (under the tongue), anterior two-thirds of the tongue and buccal mucosa (inside the cheek)

These cancers are more aggressive than lip cancers, growing and spreading more rapidly, and the enlargement of lymph nodes containing secondary spread of cancer is rather common.

The cancer is usually first noticed as an ulcer or a lump, sometimes by a dentist, before the patient has become aware of any problem. Other common features are bleeding or localised soreness. Such cancers tend to be on the surface at first but soon invade locally, with firm thickness and induration surrounding the lump or ulcer. They usually become quite tender. Diagnosis is confirmed by taking a small piece of tissue as a biopsy for examination under the microscope.

Most of these cancers are treated by surgical excision or radiotherapy. Lymph nodes are best treated by surgical excision of all lymph nodes in the region (block dissection).

For larger cancers in the floor of the mouth, anterior two-thirds of the tongue and possibly in the cheek, treatment by a combination of chemotherapy and radiotherapy may be required. By these simultaneous combined treatments, or alternatively if the chemotherapy can be given by intra-arterial infusion, cures can now be achieved in patients with advanced cancers that until recently were considered incurable or curable only by the most radical surgery. Such treatments require special skills, equipment and experience and should only be carried out in specialist cancer centres.

Cancers in the posterior third of the tongue, tonsillar region and pharynx

People with these cancers may present with an ulcer, a lump in the throat or tongue, or sometimes with a constant sore throat that has not responded to medical treatment, including antibiotics. Sometimes patients will first notice a lump in the side of the neck, which is an enlarged hard lymph node containing secondary cancer. Diagnosis may appear to be obvious but must be confirmed by biopsy.

Except for small cancers in this region, most are not curable by surgery. Radiotherapy is likely to cure only small cancers, although it may offer good temporary palliation to people with large cancers.

Most people with these cancers do not visit a doctor or clinic until the cancer is advanced and the chances of cure by surgery or radiotherapy are not good. Most will be heavy smokers, and many will also be heavy alcohol drinkers. They may not notice the symptoms until the cancers are at a late stage. In any case, these cancers are aggressive and tend to grow and invade locally and spread into lymph nodes on one or both sides of the neck at a relatively early stage.

Radical surgery will cure some of these patients, but cure is more likely to result from combined chemotherapy and radiotherapy, with or without following surgery. For incurable cancers combined therapy will at least give good palliation to the majority. The chemotherapy and radiotherapy may be given simultaneously as chemo/radiotherapy or may be given over a more prolonged period – first giving the chemotherapy, preferably by intra-arterial infusion, followed later by radiotherapy. Special experience, skills and facilities are required for these procedures, so the most appropriate treatment will depend on the skills and experience of the treatment team (see Section 2).

Cancers of the post-nasal space (back of the nose)

These cancers are most common in adult Chinese people, especially those from the Guangdong province of China.

Immigrant descendants of these people have an increased incidence of this cancer, even though they may never have lived in China.

Blood tests show that this cancer is most common in people who have been infected with the Epstein-Barr virus: their blood usually has a high level of Epstein-Barr-virus antibodies. If the Epstein-Barr test is high before treatment and returns to normal after treatment, it indicates that treatment has been successful and the patient has probably been cured.

Symptoms and signs

People with post-nasal-space cancer may present with symptoms of a blocked nose and nasal or post-nasal discharge of mucus, pus or bloodstained material. Alternatively, they sometimes first notice a lump in the side of the neck. The lump is due to secondary cancer in a lymph node. Sometimes lymph nodes on both sides of the neck are involved.

The cancer may sometimes be seen with a mirror in the back of the throat, but diagnosis is made by taking a biopsy from the back of the nose or sometimes by removing an enlarged lymph node from the neck for pathological examination.

Occasionally the cancer invades bones at the base of the skull or the cranial nerves that pass from the brain through the base of the skull and into the neck. CT or MRI scans may be taken to look for evidence of bone involvement.

Treatment

Cancer in the back of the nose is not accessible to surgery. It is usually treated by radiotherapy, with better than a 50% chance of cure provided the cancer has not spread into lymph nodes in the neck or invaded bone behind the nose at the base of the skull. If lymph nodes in the neck are involved, the chance of cure by radiotherapy alone is reduced (possibly to only 30–40%) and considerably lower if nodes on both sides of the neck are involved. However, combined integrated chemotherapy and radiotherapy (see Section 2) has improved the outcome in advanced cancers, especially if lymph nodes are involved.

If bone at the base of the skull is invaded by cancer, the chance of cure by any means is poor.

Cancer of the larynx

Cancer of the larynx is most common in smokers, especially smokers who are also heavy drinkers. It is more common in men than women. The most common site is on a vocal cord, which can cause hoarseness or change in the voice when the cancer is small and is therefore usually diagnosed early. They can be seen and biopsied through a laryngoscope. If treated early, either by radiotherapy or by surgery (in which the cord is removed), the results of treatment are good, with a 90% cure rate.

If neglected until the cancer has grown from the vocal cord into surrounding tissues, however, the chances of cure by simple surgery or radiotherapy are much reduced.

For the more advanced laryngeal cancers that have spread to the walls of the larynx or spread into lymph nodes in the neck, or cancers that have recurred after previous radiotherapy, the best chance of cure is by radical surgery in which the larynx is removed, possibly together with all draining lymph nodes (an operation called a radical laryngectomy).

Cancers in the larynx that develop above or below the vocal cords are usually more advanced when they are first diagnosed than cancers on a vocal cord. They also tend to be more aggressive and for this reason are often treated by combined radiotherapy and laryngectomy or even combined chemo/radio-therapy and laryngectomy.

After removal of the larynx, the chance of cure is reasonably good, but the patient (usually a male) is left with an opening in his windpipe in the lower neck (a tracheotomy). Without a larynx he cannot speak normally, but most patients learn a form of oesophageal speech. By this method they can be taught to swallow air and regurgitate air from the stomach to make sounds and words. Alternatively, a mechanical vibrator powered by a small battery can be applied to the throat muscles to make speech that sounds rather like the artificial voice of a robot or computer.

The Lost Cords club is a group for people who have lost their larynx and support each other in learning to speak and in other social, health and mechanical problems. As with mastectomy groups (for women who have had a breast removed) and colostomy groups (for patients with a colostomy), there are branches in many big cities. The group helps people who have had a laryngectomy to adjust to their changed circumstances. It also helps patients learn to speak so that they can live a relatively normal life again.

Salivary-gland cancers

The salivary glands are located about the mouth and secrete saliva into the mouth to prepare food for digestion. There are three major and many minor salivary glands on each side of the face.

The largest salivary gland is the parotid gland, situated partly in front of and below the ear and behind the jaw. This is the salivary gland in which both benign and malignant tumours develop most commonly. The second-largest major salivary gland is the submandibular gland under the jaw, and the third major salivary gland is the sublingual gland in the floor of the mouth under the tongue. The many small minor salivary glands are in the mucous membrane (lining) of the tongue, lips, palate, cheek and pharynx.

Cancers of the salivary glands are usually first noticed as a lump, most commonly just in front of or below the ear. As the cancer enlarges, it may invade and destroy the important facial nerve, which passes through the parotid gland. Damage to the facial nerve causes weakness of the muscles of that side of the face, resulting in an inability to close the eye or move the corner of the mouth properly. There may be obvious loss of facial expression due to paralysis of the muscles on that side of the face. These cancers most often develop in middle-aged or older adults. They enlarge locally and tend to spread to local lymph nodes in front of the ear and in the upper part of the neck. Occasionally cancers develop from a pre-existing benign tumour in the parotid gland that may have been present for years, known as a mixed parotid tumour or pleomorphic adenoma.

Treatment of cancers of the parotid gland is usually by removal through a surgical operation. With small cancers it may be possible to save the facial nerve, but with larger cancers it is likely that the facial nerve will be involved and will need to be removed. If lymph nodes are enlarged, they are usually removed in the same block of tissue with the parotid gland. Post-operative radiotherapy is often given in view of the risk of local recurrence of these cancers.

Cancers in the submandibular and sublingual salivary glands are not common, but when present they tend to spread rapidly to lymph nodes and are best treated by surgical excision of the whole of the gland, together with any involved lymph nodes. Salivary-gland cancers also occasionally occur in the minor salivary glands, either in the tongue, in the cheeks, lips or elsewhere about the mouth. Wide surgical excision is required for treatment as the chances of local recurrence are high unless a lot of tissue around the lump is removed. If there is any doubt that the cancer has been totally removed, then radiotherapy may also be given after the operation.

Chemotherapy in the treatment of salivary-gland cancers has

generally not been of benefit, although success has been reported in treating locally aggressive cancers using regional-induction chemotherapy before surgery.

Cancer of the thyroid gland

The thyroid gland lies across the lower part of the neck, with one lobe on either side of the trachea (or windpipe) and on the lower part of the larynx (voice box). The thyroid gland uses iodine to make a hormone called thyroxine, which is essential for normal body function.

Enlargement of the thyroid gland is called a goitre, and multiple cysts and other lumps may develop in some goitres. This process is usually due to a shortage of iodine in the food. A lumpy goitre is known as a multinodular goitre.

Occasionally one of the lumps in a multinodular goitre will become malignant and form a cancer, but more often a cancer develops as a single lump in an otherwise apparently normal thyroid gland.

Thus cancer of the thyroid is usually first noticed as a single lump in the thyroid gland, most often just to one side of the midline in the lower part of the neck. It may occasionally develop in a goitre as one lump that enlarges and becomes more obvious and hard.

Investigations

An isotope scan is a useful investigation for thyroid cancer. A scan of the thyroid is taken after injection of a very small dose of radioactive iodine into a vein (see Section 2) and will usually show a 'cold nodule', that is, the part of the thyroid gland that has been replaced by cancer does not concentrate the iodine and appears clear on the scan. However, cysts and some other lumps also show up as 'cold nodules'. To make a diagnosis, the lump should be biopsied. This may sometimes be done by needle aspiration of fluid or cells from the lump, but the diagnosis is more certain if the lump is surgically excised and examined under a microscope. Frozen-section examination (see Section 2) may then allow the surgeon to proceed with further surgery immediately if the lump proves to be a cancer.

There are three main types of thyroid cancer.

The most common of the thyroid cancers (more than 60%) is the least malignant. This is called a papillary cancer and occurs three times more commonly in women than in men. This cancer often occurs in young people, occasionally teenagers or even children.

Papillary cancer may be present in different parts of the thyroid gland at the same time and may spread to nearby draining lymph nodes, but it usually does not spread further until very late in the disease. For this reason removal of the whole of the thyroid gland, together with any enlarged lymph nodes, will usually cure the patient. After total removal of the thyroid gland the patient must take thyroxine tablets by mouth.

The second most common type of thyroid cancer tends to affect adults of middle age and is called follicular cancer. It, too, usually presents as a lump in the thyroid gland and is usually not diagnosed with certainty until the lump has been removed surgically and examined under the microscope.

These cancers tend to be present in one lobe of the thyroid gland only and have a greater tendency to spread by the bloodstream to bone, lungs or liver rather than by lymphatics to lymph nodes. These cancers often more closely resemble normal thyroid tissue than do the other thyroid cancers, and although they usually appear as 'cold nodules' (areas of no function) in radio-iodine scans, they may sometimes scan as normal thyroid tissue or even rarely as hyperactive 'hot nodules' (areas with increased thyroid function).

Because of their tendency to involve one lobe of the thyroid gland only, they are usually treated by removal of the involved half of the thyroid gland, leaving the other half to carry out normal thyroid function and production of thyroxine.

Secondary cancers may be treated by surgical excision (if in lymph nodes), by radiotherapy or by radioactive iodine treatment. Chemotherapy is also sometimes used in the treatment of secondary cancers.

The third broad type of thyroid cancer is anaplastic cancer. As this is the most dangerous form of thyroid cancer, it is fortunate that it is also the least common. It tends to affect older people and may grow rapidly, presenting as an enlarging lump or enlarging swelling of the whole of the thyroid gland. It may press on the trachea (windpipe) and make breathing difficult. This cancer is virtually incurable by surgery and is best palliated by radiotherapy or sometimes chemotherapy.

The thyroid gland is occasionally the site of other primary malignant cancers, such as medullary cancer, lymphoma, sarcoma or even secondary cancers, but these are uncommon forms of thyroid malignancy.

CANCERS OF THE FEMALE SEXUAL ORGANS

Cancer of the uterus

There are two distinct types of cancer of the uterus: squamous-cell carcinoma (SCC) of the cervix (neck of uterus) and adenocarcinoma of the lining of the body of the uterus. SCC of the cervix is more common.

Cancer of the cervix

This cancer is most common in women who have had sexual activity with multiple partners starting early in life. Infection with a sexually transmitted virus, the human papilloma virus (HPV), is the major cause. It is also more common in women who have had several children, particularly if erosions and inflammation of the cervix resulted from the multiple pregnancies.

The earliest changes associated with this cancer are most frequently present in women between the ages of 30 and 40. Usually at this age there are no symptoms, but there may be a little blood-staining from the vagina between periods, especially after intercourse.

Cancers of the cervix tend to develop slowly but can usually be detected by routine cervical-screening examination (the Papanicolaou or cervical-smear test described in Section 2), in which abnormal (dysplastic) or frankly malignant cells may be found. A cervical-smear test is recommended at least every second year for all women or more frequently if there has been any suggestion of a special risk, to detect these cancers early and at a very curable stage.

Sometimes the cancers cannot be seen on visual examination of the cervix, but at other times a cancer may be seen as an eroded, reddish, ulcerated or possibly bleeding lesion. A biopsy is taken for pathological examination to confirm the diagnosis.

Very small early cancers may be treated by surgical removal of the cervix only, especially in women who wish to have more babies. Larger invasive cancers are best treated by removal of the uterus (total hysterectomy).

If cancer of the cervix is not diagnosed until it is more advanced, there is a risk that it may have spread to lymph nodes, especially the lymph nodes in the pelvis. This situation is more likely to be found in women of more than 40 years of age who have not had regular cervical-smear tests. These women often complain of some bleeding and discharge between periods. If an advanced, ulcerating or fungating cancer is present, it should be obvious on examination of the cervix. Surrounding tissues, such as the ureters (the tubes that pass urine from the kidneys to the bladder) or the rectum, may become involved, as well as the local draining lymph nodes in the pelvis. Such advanced cancers are usually treated by combination chemo/radiotherapy, possibly followed by surgery.

A truly major advance has been the development of a vaccine against HPV, which may eventually eradicate most cancers of the cervix in the way that smallpox and polio have been eradicated. Some people may experience a negative reaction, such as fainting, but this is also the case with many other vaccinations. In Australia it has become readily available at no cost for teenage girls and women up to 26 years of age, and is now also available for older women at their own expense.

Cancer of the body of the uterus (endometrial cancer)

Endometrial cancers tend to occur in older women, usually after menopause. It is believed that changes in female sex hormones, and especially an imbalance of hormones, may contribute to the development of these cancers.

The most common feature is post-menopausal bleeding and blood-stained discharge. The uterus is usually found to be enlarged. To make a diagnosis, the doctor performs a curettage and sends the specimens removed for microscopic examination.

Treatment of cancer of the body of the uterus is usually by complete removal of the uterus (total hysterectomy), with the removal of ovaries as well as lymph nodes in the pelvis. For advanced cancers radiotherapy is often given first as well.

As with most cancers, treatment at an early stage will allow good results, but for more advanced cancers the results of treatment are often disappointing.

If endometrial cancer has spread to other tissues or organs, it will often respond to hormone treatment (large-dose progesterone therapy), but a long-term cure is unlikely. Studies are being made of combined integrated treatment using chemotherapy first as 'induction' treatment, followed by radiotherapy and/or surgery (see Section 2).

Choriocarcinoma

Although a choriocarcinoma starts and grows in the uterus, it is not strictly a cancer of the uterus. A choriocarcinoma is best considered as a cancer of an abnormal pregnancy.

After conception an abnormal growth of tissue very occasionally develops instead of a normal foetus and placenta. If the foetus does not develop and the placenta grows as a group of cyst-like structures, something like a bunch of grapes, this is called a hydatidiform mole.

Sometimes the cells of a hydatidiform mole develop into an invasive cancer that is called a choriocarcinoma. Occasionally choriocarcinoma will develop in association with a foetus, usually abnormal, which is aborted spontaneously, or even with an otherwise normal pregnancy. However, most are in association with a hydatidiform mole, usually in women over 40 years of age.

In the past, choriocarcinoma spread widely and rapidly through the mother's body and was a fatal form of cancer. Now the condition is treated by emptying the uterus of its contents (a curette) and giving combination chemotherapy. This is one of the success stories of modern chemotherapy, as choriocarcinoma was almost 100% fatal about 30 years ago but is now curable in 80% or more of cases.

Cancer of the ovary

The ovaries are the source of a greater variety of tumours, both benign and malignant, than any other organ. This is probably because of the nature of the ovaries as organs, with their function of undergoing monthly cyclic changes to produce eggs or ova for potential development into the new tissues of a foetus. They may also produce tumours that excrete hormones that may affect body development and function.

Cancers of the ovary may be solid, cystic or contain a mixture of solid and cystic elements. They tend to cause no symptoms early in their development, because they can easily grow to a large size in the pelvic/abdominal cavity without interfering with other structures, and so are often quite advanced when first diagnosed.

Symptoms and signs

When they have reached a certain size, cancers of the ovary usually cause a swelling in the pelvis and lower abdomen. The swelling may have been noticed by the patient or may be found on examination by a doctor. They may also sometimes cause local discomfort or pain. If they produce hormones, the first evidence may be due to hormonal changes such as premature cessation of menstruation and loss of feminine features, with a development of male characteristics such as growth of hair on the face or deepening of the voice. Sometimes generalised abdominal swelling may also be noticed, due either to a huge tumour or to fluid in the abdominal cavity (ascites).

Any rapidly enlarging swelling on an ovary, especially if it is solid or contains a mixture of cystic and solid elements, must be regarded with suspicion as likely to be malignant.

Investigations

A doctor will carry out an examination of the pelvis and pelvic structures by examining the lower abdomen, the vagina and rectum, but if this examination is not adequate the patient may be admitted to hospital for examination under a general anaesthetic.

Abdominal X-rays or CT scans may help, but ultrasound examination is usually the most helpful and the least harmful examination, especially in young women.

Laparoscopy or culdoscopy (see Section 2) may allow the surgeon or gynaecologist to see the contents of the pelvis, especially the ovaries.

Usually the diagnosis of cancer cannot be established with certainty until an operation (laparoscopy or laparotomy) has been carried out and a biopsy specimen of any suspicious lesion has been examined under the microscope.

Treatment

The best treatment of ovarian cancer is by the surgical removal of the ovaries. As the other ovary and sometimes other pelvic organs may also contain cancer, it is usual to remove both ovaries as well as the uterus and fallopian tubes and any other involved tissue. The operation may be followed by radiotherapy to the pelvis and abdomen. Often advanced tumours are removed as much as possible (cyto-reductive surgery) and the patient is then treated with a combination of chemotherapy drugs. This can frequently lead to a worthwhile remission. The drugs used are commonly of the platinum and taxol classes in combination.

Prevention

As cancers sometimes develop from benign tumours of the ovary and the ovaries have little function in post-menopausal women, it is usually advisable to remove both ovaries of women over 40 when treating a benign ovarian tumour. Gynaecologists also often advise removal of ovaries as a preventive measure when they perform hysterectomy (removal of the uterus) in women over the age of 40.

The ovaries are commonly a site for the development of secondary cancer from a primary cancer elsewhere. Cancer of the breast, stomach and bowel, and melanoma frequently spread to ovaries. These are removed if there is no apparent cancer anywhere else; otherwise treatment given will depend upon the best treatment for the type of cancer concerned and where it came from.

Cancer of the vulva

Like cancer of the anus, cancer of the vulva is a rather aggressive form of skin cancer, usually of the SCC type. Most occur in women of post-menopausal age. This cancer is often preceded by a long history of irritation or discomfort of the vulva, possibly with a local bloodstained discharge. There may be a pre-malignant condition of leukoplakia or a chronic rash. Previous infection with the sexually transmitted HPV may be responsible for some cases.

In the more advanced disease there may be an ulcer, a lump or a cauliflower-like growth. Spread to lymph nodes in one or both groins is likely to be present in about half of the patients.

Diagnosis is established by biopsy, and treatment is usually by wide and radical surgical excision, most often with satisfactory results, with most patients being cured. Pre-malignant conditions are also best treated by surgical excision to prevent cancer developing.

For very advanced cases radiotherapy offers palliative relief. Combination chemo/radiotherapy is used in some cases before or after surgery.

CANCER OF THE MALE SEXUAL ORGANS

Cancer of the testis

Testicular tumours are relatively rare, but when they do occur they are almost always malignant. Most occur in young adult males between the ages of 20 and 40.

There are no known causes of testicular cancer, apart from

those cancers occurring in testes that have not descended into the scrotum from the abdomen at birth. If the testes are not present in the scrotum of infant boys, a surgical operation may be required to place the testes in their normal position. This may reduce the risk of development of testis cancer later in life, some time after puberty.

There are two main types of testicular cancer: seminoma and non-seminoma (also known as teratoma).

Seminoma is composed of a more or less uniform type of cell derived from the precursors of sperm cells.

Non-seminomas may have complex mixtures of pathological subtypes that are apparently more closely related to primitive pregnancy-like cells (e.g. yolk-sac, embryonal or chorio-carcinoma types).

Symptoms and signs

Cancer of the testis is usually found as a painless and non-tender swelling of a testis. Only rarely is the swelling tender or painful. Occasionally swelling is not seen in the testis until there is evidence of the metastatic spread of the testicular cancer. These metastases may be noticed as a mass of enlarged and sometimes tender lymph nodes in the abdomen, enlarged lymph nodes in the neck (usually the left side) or as secondary cancers in lungs seen in a chest X-ray. Occasionally the first evidence of a testicular cancer may be the swelling of a man's breasts due to changes in his hormones. In other patients the first evidence may be of general debility, anorexia (loss of appetite) and weight loss.

Investigations

If a swelling of a testis is likely to be cancer, investigations are carried out to look for evidence of secondary spread. CT scans, described in Section 2, may be helpful in detecting any enlarged lymph nodes in the abdomen and chest or involvement of the liver.

To confirm a diagnosis of cancer the operation of orchidectomy (removal of the testis) is carried out. The incision is carried out in the groin and the entire testis and cancer are removed from the scrotum. It is important also to have a blood sample sent to pathology for measurement of the tumour markers that are specific to testicular cancers, b-hCG and alpha-feto-protein. If these tumour markers are elevated, a fall in their levels after surgery can indicate that there is no metastatic spread and that the whole cancer has been successfully removed.

Treatment

Cancer of a testis is first treated by surgical removal of the testis.

For patients with seminoma and no evidence of spread after CT scans a simple course of radiotherapy to the draining lymph nodes in the abdomen is given as adjuvant treatment.

A careful follow-up watch is kept on patients with non-seminoma-type tumours and no evidence of spread detected in the follow-up blood tests and CT scans. However, even if the disease recurs or is widespread at diagnosis the vast majority of patients can be cured with combination chemotherapy. The drug cisplatinum is used, and it has been responsible for the dramatic improvement in outcome.

It is possible to subsequently lead a normal sex life and to father children with only one testis.

Cancer of the prostate

Cancer of the prostate is uncommon before the age of 50, but in Western societies it is the most common cancer in men over 65 and is increasing in incidence.

Its cause is unknown, but its association with old age is illustrated by the fact that more than 75% of men over the age of 90 have microscopic evidence of at least early prostate cancer. This cancer is less common in Asian countries. It is likely that the Western diet, high in animal products, plays a significant part in causing prostate cancer.

Recent studies have indicated that diets with a high content of legumes such as soybeans may be protective. These contain naturally occurring plant hormones (phytoestrogens) that may play a part in cancer prevention.

Symptoms and signs

The most common symptom of prostatic cancer is difficulty in passing urine. Non-malignant enlargement of the prostate (benign prostatic hypertrophy or BPH) is most often the cause of urinary difficulty, but prostate cancer is also a common cause, especially in older men.

Sometimes the first evidence of cancer of the prostate can be symptoms due to metastatic cancer either in the bone (causing pain or fractures) or in the liver. Secondary cancers in the lower vertebral column (back bone) or pelvis may cause pressure on a sciatic nerve that passes into the leg, causing severe pain in the back and leg called sciatica. Sciatica is more often caused by other conditions, but occasionally it is the first evidence of a cancer of the prostate.

Investigations

The prostate gland can be felt by a doctor in a PR (per rectal) examination. That is, a gloved finger is passed through the anus into the rectum and the prostate gland can be felt in front of the finger. Cancer in the prostate feels like a hard lump in the prostate, or sometimes the whole of the gland may feel hard and rigid.

CT studies will show the size and extent of the prostate, but ultrasound studies taken through the rectum will more precisely show any lumps or nodules in the prostate that may be a cancer. A biopsy may be taken with a needle on a spring-loaded gun directed into the prostate by ultrasound via the rectum.

X-rays will be taken for evidence of secondary spread into bones. These usually show up as sclerotic (dense white) areas in the bone. Chest X-rays may show evidence of secondary cancers in the lungs, in lymph nodes in the chest or even in the ribs. Isotope bone scans are also valuable in showing evidence of secondary bone cancer.

Blood studies may show evidence of anaemia due to secondary bone cancer destroying the blood-forming cells in bone marrow. Obstruction by the cancer of the flow of urine may cause infection in the bladder and possibly in the kidneys.

The urine and blood are examined for evidence of infection in urine and for evidence of damage to the kidneys.

In recent years a blood test, the prostate specific antigen (PSA) screening test, has been developed to indicate whether there is likely to be an abnormality in the prostate. This is a special immunological test that is now commonly used in men over the age of 50 to help find those with early prostate cancer who might be effectively treated by operation. A raised PSA level does not necessarily indicate that cancer is present, but it does indicate the need for further investigations, possibly including ultrasound study and biopsies. It may be highly elevated in men with metastatic spread to bone.

Treatment and treatment controversies

There is considerable controversy in regard to both the value of screening tests and the actual treatment of prostate cancer. The PSA screening test has led to the diagnosis of prostate cancer in increasing numbers of middle-aged and elderly males. Yet even if a biopsy diagnosis of cancer is confirmed, it is estimated that only about one in four of those cancers will grow in a malignant fashion and spread to tissues beyond the prostate in such a way that it is likely to cause the patient's death. There is as yet no definite way of identifying those cancers that are likely to spread. Most prostate cancers are slow growing and even after many years may show no evidence of spread, but some will spread to such places as lungs, liver and especially to bones, where they are likely to form painful secondaries and lead to the death of the patient.

Appropriate treatment of early prostate cancer will cure most patients, but all treatments have serious side effects, and it is not entirely possible at this stage to determine which patients will benefit from treatment and who might just as well be left without treatment.

The most distressing treatment side effect is impotence. This occurs in 50% or more of patients, whether treated by total prostatectomy (surgical removal of the whole prostate gland) or by radiotherapy. Treatments available at present are often effective for impotence resulting from prostatectomy, but when hormone treatment is used to treat metastatic disease, either by giving anti-testosterone medication or by orchidectomy (castration) or both, impotence is virtually inevitable.

Although controversial, the following are standard treatments that should be considered and discussed between a patient and his medical advisors.

For small cancers apparently confined to the prostate, total surgical removal of the prostate gland, and if necessary with removal of adjacent lymph nodes, should result in cure. This may be the best treatment for men who are reasonably young and fit with an otherwise long life expectancy.

Alternatively, obstruction to the flow of urine may be relieved by a TUR (trans-urethral resection), in which an instrument (resectoscope) is passed into the urethra through the penis and some of the enlarged prostate is cut away to relieve obstruction. Specimens of the tissue are sent for microscopic examination.

Cancer of the prostate will often respond to radiotherapy, which is often used to treat both primary prostate cancer and a limited number of painful secondary deposits in bone. If radiotherapy is used to treat the primary cancer, it can be given as a conventional external beam or as radioactive pellets actually inserted into the prostate. This is called brachytherapy. Modern techniques of brachytherapy can now produce equally good results to surgery.

The male hormone testosterone stimulates prostate cancer, so anti-testosterone treatment is also used, especially for more widespread cancer. Patients with metastatic prostate cancer are often given effective palliative relief by treatment with such drugs. The drugs used either antagonise the action of testosterone or inhibit its synthesis. An alternative treatment likely to give similar response is to remove the source of male hormones, the testes (bilateral orchidectomy).

Prostate cancer will respond to treatment with some cytotoxic agents, but these are normally only used in patients whose advanced cancer no longer responds to hormone management. Excellent improvements in quality of life can be obtained when relatively non-toxic forms of chemotherapy are used, often in combination with cortisone-like drugs such as prednisone.

CANCERS OF THE BLADDER AND KIDNEYS
Bladder cancer
Although rare today, more than a century ago bladder cancer

was found to be increased in industrial workers exposed to aniline dyes and rubber manufacturing.

Smokers have about a threefold increased risk of contracting bladder cancer. It is also more common in the Nile valley in Egypt, where parasitic diseases (schistosomiasis) infecting the bladder start an inflammatory process that can develop into malignancy. Cancer may also develop in a benign cauliflower-like tumour of the bladder known as a papilloma. Some patients have several small papillomas in the bladder wall, and any one of these can change to a cancer if not treated.

The most common symptom of bladder cancer is blood in the urine (haematuria). The blood may be intermittent at first but becomes more constant as the cancer grows and invades the bladder wall. At a later stage there may be discomfort in passing urine (dysuria) and symptoms of bladder infection (cystitis), increased frequency of passing urine, and burning and pain. Sometimes a ureter (the tube through which urine passes from the kidney to the bladder) may become obstructed by the growth and may cause pain in the loins due to back pressure on the kidney.

After losing blood in the urine for some time, anaemia may develop and symptoms of anaemia (pallor, tiredness, palpitations, etc.) may be noticed.

Investigations

The urine is examined for blood and may also be examined for cancer cells. Excretory urograms (IVP X-rays, described in Section 2) may show a filling defect or lump in the bladder. They may also show evidence of obstruction to a ureter if this is present. A CT scan may reveal a lump in the bladder wall.

The critical investigation, however, is cystoscopy. The flexible fibre-optic cystoscope (discussed in Section 2) is passed into the bladder through the urethra (the tube for passage of urine from the bladder), usually under general anaesthesia. The inside of the bladder is then examined by the doctor. A small piece of any suspected cancer together with a small piece of adjacent bladder wall is taken as a biopsy for microscopic examination.

Types of bladder cancer (pathology)

There are various degrees of bladder tumours, ranging from a single benign cauliflower-like papilloma to an invasive, rigid, ulcerated and thickened cancer. Between these extremes there may be several papillomata (small warts or cauliflower-like growths), one or more of which may show signs of early malignancy, or there may be a malignant lump in the bladder wall. Bladder cancers tend to remain confined to the bladder wall for a long time before they spread. After a time, however, bladder cancers may involve the whole thickness of the bladder wall and even invade the rectum or other organs nearby in the pelvis. They may also spread to nearby lymph nodes and subsequently to lungs and other organs.

Treatment

Small papillomata of the bladder are usually treated by burning them off with an instrument called an electro-cautery, which is used through a cystoscope, or simply resected. The patient is cystoscoped regularly afterwards in case the tumour recurs.

For larger papillomas or early invasive cancers treatment by radiotherapy or surgical excision, or a combination of both radiotherapy and surgical excision, may offer good prospects of cure. Subsequent instillation of a modified bacteria (BCG) into the bladder can induce an immune response retarding tumour regrowth.

For more advanced cancers it may be necessary to operate to remove the whole of the bladder (total cystectomy). A new type of bladder is then usually made by the surgeon from a part of the bowel.

When cure by surgery is not possible, palliative radiotherapy may give relief. Chemotherapy has a limited place in the treatment of bladder cancer but can offer palliation in some patients with metastatic cancer.

Cancers of the kidney

Kidney cancers are not common, but there are three well-recognised types. The Wilms' tumour or nephroblastoma occurs in children. In adults kidney cancers are either the adenocarcinoma (sometimes called hypernephroma or Grawitz tumour) or carcinoma of the renal pelvis.

Wilms' tumour (nephroblastoma)

Wilms' tumour is usually found in children of less than four years of age and can even be present at birth. Although in most cases only one kidney is affected, occasionally it is bilateral (i.e. present in both kidneys). This cancer is most commonly found as a lump in the loin of an infant. It may cause the child to be in general poor health, with a fever, anaemia or sometimes blood in the urine. It may spread to nearby lymph nodes or into the large veins. From these veins cancer cells may be carried by the blood to the lungs, where secondary growths may develop.

Adenocarcinoma (Grawitz tumour or hypernephroma)

This is the most common type of kidney cancer and is usually seen in adults of middle age or older. The first symptom is usually the passage of blood in the urine, most often not associated with pain. (Passing of blood in the urine with pain in the loin is more likely to be caused by a kidney stone.) There may be a fever, or a lump may be felt in the loin, or sometimes there is localised pain. This cancer may spread into nearby lymph nodes but commonly grows into the large renal vein (the vein taking blood from the kidney) and may spread by the bloodstream into the lungs, liver or bones. Sometimes the first evidence of this cancer is the presence of secondary cancers in a lung or in one or more bones.

Adult smokers have a twofold to threefold increase in the incidence of kidney cancers.

Carcinoma of the renal pelvis

Carcinoma of the renal pelvis is rather like cancer of the bladder and behaves in a similar manner. The first sign is usually blood in the urine. This cancer sometimes develops as a reaction to a stone present in the kidney for a long time.

Investigations for kidney cancers

X-rays of the abdomen may show an enlarged kidney. Excretory urograms (IVP), CT scans, ultrasound and arteriography (see Section 2) are all useful investigations to help diagnose a tumour in a kidney. They will also help determine whether a kidney lump is solid and likely to be cancer or a fluid-filled cyst and probably not malignant.

Other investigations include examination of the urine for blood or malignant cells and X-rays of the lungs for evidence of secondary cancer. If there is evidence of swelling or painful areas in bones, these will be X-rayed and bone scans may be arranged to look for evidence of secondary bone cancers.

Treatment

Cancer of a kidney is best treated by surgical operation to remove the kidney (nephrectomy).

For Wilms' tumour (nephroblastoma) in children results are much better if radiotherapy and chemotherapy are used in combination with surgical removal of the kidney.

For adenocarcinoma surgical treatment (removal of the kidney) is the only likely cure for a patient. Radiotherapy and chemotherapy may be used as palliative treatment in advanced cases, but results have been disappointing. Sometimes these cancers will show a temporary response to male or female hormones. Adenocarcinoma of the kidney can sometimes spread to a lung as a single secondary, and this can sometimes be cured by an operation removing the part of the lung containing the metastasis. Similarly, patients who have only a few slow-growing metastases can have very long-lasting positive responses to intensive radiotherapy.

For cancer of the renal pelvis best results are achieved if the kidney is removed together with the whole of the ureter and a small part of the bladder as small seedlings of this cancer sometimes grow in the ureter between the kidney and the bladder. The new generations of small-molecule signal-inhibiting targeted drugs, such as Glivec, which is especially effective in treating chronic myeloid leukaemia, are showing encouraging results in clinical trials, but as yet they are not generally available.

CANCERS OF THE BRAIN

Although most brain cancers occur in people over the age of 45 with a peak incidence between 60 and 70, the brain is also one of the more common sites for primary cancer in children and young adults.

There are two groups of cells in the brain that may form tumours: the glial cells (or true brain cells), from which most of the malignant tumours (cancers) develop; and the non-glial cells or supporting cells (such as cells of the meninges covering the brain or cells of the sheaths surrounding nerves), from which develop the majority of non-malignant (benign) tumours.

Cancers that arise from true brain cells or glial cells are called gliomas. There are a number of different types of gliomas, which range from the more slow-growing types called astrocytoma or oligodendroglioma to more rapid and highly malignant types called medulloblastoma or glioblastoma multiforme. These different types of glioma tend to occur in different parts of the brain in children and adults. They also have other differences: the medulloblastomas (more commonly seen in young people) are usually highly radio-sensitive and are sometimes cured by radiotherapy, but other types are less radio-sensitive, if at all.

Symptoms and signs

Brain cancers tend to cause two types of clinical features:

- general features due to generalised pressure on the brain;
- focal or local features due to pressure or interference by the tumour on parts of the brain or nerves near the tumour.

The common general features of cancer in the brain are due to pressure on and swelling of the brain as a whole. This causes headaches, nausea, vomiting and disturbances of vision due to papilloedema (swelling of the optic nerve at the back of the eye). Other features may include listlessness, tiredness and personality change. The sufferer may progressively withdraw from social contact and gradually become confused and stuporous, and may lapse into coma. In young children the increased pressure may cause the head to enlarge, and hydrocephalus (so-called 'water on the brain') may develop.

It should be noted that in children, convulsions or fitting are most often caused by a fever or other less serious problems. Fitting alone is rarely caused by cancer in children. In an adult with no previous history of epilepsy, injury or fitting from another known cause, however, the sudden onset of a fitting attack may be the first sign of a brain tumour.

Focal features are due to the cancer's interference with the function of a local region of brain. These features will depend upon the site of the tumour. In one place it may be interference with speech, in another it may be loss of movement of an arm or leg and in another it may be loss of feeling or sensation of a part of the body. Tumours in other places may cause local twitching or focal fitting with different sensations, such as sensation of smell or visual hallucinations like the flickering of lights. In other areas tumours may cause disorders of balance, clumsy movement or interference with cranial nerves (the nerves that leave the brain), such as the optic nerves for vision, the nerves that move the eyeball or the facial nerves that move the muscles of the side of the face.

Investigations

The CT and MRI scans have revolutionised investigations for brain tumours. Before these scans were invented, cerebral arteriography (X-rays of arteries supplying the brain), radio-isotope scans and air encephalograms (see Section 2) were used almost routinely, together with a number of other investigations such as the EEG (electroencephalogram), which records brainwave activity. Nowadays, however, the MRI scan in particular usually supplies most of the information that could be obtained by these older investigations and even more precisely. Angiography may still give added information, particularly concerning the accumulation of new blood vessels in the cancer that supply it with blood.

Treatment

Most benign cerebral tumours can be cured by surgical removal, but malignant tumours (brain cancers) are not often curable. For this reason it is vital to determine – usually at operation – whether a tumour in the brain is benign or malignant (cancer). If malignant, it is also important to determine the type of malignancy, as the outlook for some types is better than others and some (such as medulloblastomas) may be curable.

Although most true brain cancers (gliomas) are not curable, most patients can be given considerable relief of symptoms by a number of means. First, certain drugs (corticosteroids) can be used to reduce pressure on the brain and so relieve headaches and other pressure symptoms. Then surgical operation can be carried out to remove most of the cancer, giving further and more prolonged relief of symptoms. Following surgery the use of radiotherapy alone will usually further improve the outlook for a period.

Recent studies have shown that the use of post-operative chemotherapy with radiotherapy has given added benefit, and some apparent cures have been reported, particularly in the case of medulloblastomas.

THE LEUKAEMIAS AND LYMPHOMAS

The leukaemias

Leukaemia is a malignant growth or cancer of blood-forming cells. Leukaemias are divided into two general types according to the kind of blood-forming cell that has become malignant: the lymphoid and myeloid leukaemias.

In lymphoid leukaemia the cells that have become malignant are the bone-marrow cells that normally make the white blood cells called lymphocytes. Lymph nodes and lymphoid tissue are usually involved and become enlarged. In myeloid leukaemia the cells in the bone marrow that normally make the other types of white blood cells (e.g. polymorphs or neutrophils) have become malignant. The spleen usually becomes involved and enlarged.

Leukaemias may be acute or chronic according to whether the disease would tend to run a rapid and fatal course (acute leukaemia) or progress more slowly (chronic leukaemia). The acuteness or chronicity is determined by the maturity of the cell types involved. Thus there are four main types of leukaemia:

- acute lymphocytic (or lymphatic) leukaemia (ALL);
- acute myeloid (or non-lymphatic) leukaemia (AML or ANLL);
- chronic lymphocytic (lymphatic) leukaemia (CLL);
- chronic myeloid (granulocytic) leukaemia (CML).

It is important to distinguish between the major types of leukaemia as they have quite distinct outlooks and respond differently to different drugs.

Leukaemia occurs throughout the world, but the incidence varies in different countries and in different races. All types of leukaemia are slightly more common in males. The Scandinavian countries and Israel have the highest incidence of leukaemia, and the lowest incidence is in Chile and Japan. In the USA the highest incidence is in Jews and the lowest is in African Americans.

The overall incidence of acute lymphocytic and acute myeloid leukaemia is about equal, but there is a distinct age difference. Acute leukaemia accounts for about half of all cancers in children, and acute lymphocytic leukaemia is the most common of all cancers in young children, with a peak incidence between the ages of two and four. The incidence of acute myeloid leukaemia increases with age.

The causes of leukaemia are not known, although some predisposing factors are recognised. The myeloid leukaemias have been linked with ionising radiation, and there is evidence that exposure of a foetus to X-rays during pregnancy is associated with a slightly increased risk of leukaemia developing later in childhood. However, there is no evidence that the normal use of diagnostic X-rays in adults is associated with leukaemia.

Excessive exposure to some chemical agents such as benzene is associated with a slightly increased risk of leukaemia. Acute myeloid leukaemia will also develop a little more often in patients who have had some other form of cancer, including Hodgkin lymphoma or cancer of the ovary.

The use of anti-cancer cytotoxic drugs, and especially the use of these drugs with radiotherapy, also slightly increases the risk of later development of leukaemia.

Familial leukaemia is rare, although some families with multiple cases of leukaemia have been reported. In general the siblings of a child with leukaemia have only a slightly higher risk of developing leukaemia, although if one identical twin develops acute leukaemia the other twin has roughly a 20% chance of developing the disease as well.

People with Down's syndrome have a 20 times greater risk of developing acute leukaemia than other people. Mothers of advancing age not only have an increased risk of having children with Down's syndrome, but their non-Down's children also have a slightly greater risk of developing acute leukaemia.

Viruses are known to cause leukaemia in some animal species, but there is no evidence that this is the case in humans.

The acute leukaemias
Symptoms and signs

The symptoms of acute leukaemia are due to replacement of the normal blood-forming cells of bone marrow by malignant leukaemic cells and infiltration (invasion) of other tissues such as the spleen, lymph nodes, tonsils and sometimes the liver, kidneys, lungs and brain.

Fever, weakness, anorexia (loss of appetite), pallor and infection are common. Infection is especially common in the region of the tonsils or anus, and the lungs may also become infected, causing pneumonia. Sometimes there is pain in bones or joints. The lymph nodes, tonsils and spleen are commonly enlarged, and sometimes the liver and kidneys are enlarged.

There may be signs of bleeding from any site but especially from the gums, the digestive tract or anus. Bleeding in the brain or from the lungs may also occur. Thromboses (clots) may also develop in veins.

Meningitis due to leukaemic cell spread into the meninges (the membranes covering the brain) frequently occurs in patients with acute lymphatic leukaemia unless it is prevented by radiotherapy or chemotherapy.

Investigations

The diagnosis of leukaemia can only be made after careful examination of blood and bone marrow. Blood is taken by a needle from a vein in the arm, and bone marrow is usually taken with a small instrument that is used to puncture a bone of the pelvis (the iliac crest). Bone-marrow biopsy is done with sedation and local anaesthesia. A pathologist then examines the blood and bone marrow for leukaemic cells and for other features of leukaemia. These may include anaemia (with a reduction in numbers of red blood cells); a reduction in the number of normal white blood cells, with an increase in abnormal white cells; and a reduction in the number of platelets (the particles that help blood-clotting).

Patients with acute myeloid leukaemia are usually found to have various abnormalities of chromosomes. Analysis of these may allow some prediction of the outcome of therapy. There may also be changes in blood chemistry, such as increased uric acid (which may be associated with features of acute gout).

Treatment

Encouraging progress has been made in recent years in treatment of the acute leukaemias.

The best opportunity to achieve the maximum cure of leukaemia is when the disease is first diagnosed, as cells that remain after the first treatment tend to develop resistance to drugs. It is therefore important that patients with acute leukaemia be immediately referred for specialist care so that the most effective treatment can be given under expert supervision from the beginning.

Chemotherapy using cytotoxic drugs and cortisone forms the basis of modern treatment. Combinations of effective cytotoxic drugs have produced the best results.

Anti-cancer drugs do not pass in high concentration into the brain. Because after a time most acute lymphatic leukaemic patients will develop the disease in the brain, injections of cytotoxic drugs are given into the meningeal space around the brain. In the case of acute myeloid leukaemia, brain involvement does not occur so often, but this treatment is given immediately if there is any sign that there may be brain or central-nervous-system involvement.

With the best current treatment methods, over 90% of children and about 80% of adults with acute lymphatic leukaemia now achieve complete remission (that is, the disease apparently disappears and the patient feels and looks well again).

With acute myeloid leukaemia good results from chemotherapy have not been as reliable. Recently, in attempts to further improve results, bone-marrow transplantation has been used effectively, especially in people aged under 40. In marrow transplantation the leukaemic cells are destroyed by big doses of chemotherapy and radiotherapy (total body irradiation). This is a dangerous procedure and is only carried out in highly expert departments. The patient is then given injections of bone marrow taken from a matched donor (with similar body cells unlikely to cause a rejection reaction). The best donor is usually a parent or a sibling. More recently bone-marrow cells can be collected from the blood after injection of a bone-marrow-stimulating hormone. This is called granulocyte colony-stimulating factor (G CSF).

Bone-marrow transplantation involves a number of risks and problems and can only be carried out by appropriately trained experts in specially equipped hospitals, but the results have been most encouraging in this otherwise fatal illness. A further encouraging development is quite new at the time of writing:

when a well-matching bone-marrow donor is not available, umbilical-cord blood has been used as an alternative, with good results in children and in some adults.

In recent years treatment with immunotherapy has been further investigated. Although major success has not as yet been achieved, there have been some interesting results that give hope for better treatments becoming available in the future.

During the acute illness there may be special problems of anaemia, lowered resistance to infection, bleeding or even clotting. These may require blood transfusion or platelet transfusion and antibiotics. Aspirin should be strictly avoided as it interferes with blood-clotting.

Chronic myeloid (granulocytic) leukaemia

Chronic myeloid leukaemia can occur at any age, but its highest incidence is between the ages of 30 and 50. Although there is no known cause in most cases, it was found that in Japan five to eight years after the atomic-bomb explosions there was an increase in both acute and chronic myeloid leukaemia.

In chronic myeloid leukaemia there is a great increase in the number of white cells in the blood. This is associated with an increase in the number of cells in bone marrow. There may also be a considerable increase in the numbers of blood platelets (the particles in blood responsible for clotting). The disease is due to a very specific chromosomal abnormality that results in a mutant form of an enzyme called a signal enzyme (tyrosine-kinase) that continuously drives cell division.

Symptoms and signs

One of the more common symptoms of chronic myeloid leukaemia is pain in the left upper abdomen due to an enlarged spleen. The spleen is usually easily felt in patients with this disease (a normal spleen cannot be felt with examining fingers). There may also be features of anaemia, tiredness, weight loss or fever. Sometimes, abnormal bruising, bleeding or clotting problems may be the first evidence of the disease.

Investigations

Blood count and a bone-marrow biopsy will usually establish the diagnosis.

Treatment

There are two phases of chronic myeloid leukaemia. The chronic phase is the least dangerous and with modern treatment may last for many months or years before the dangerous acute phase takes over.

During the chronic phase the disease can now be kept under good control and possibly cured in some individuals with the drug Glivec. This is a drug form of the enzyme (called a small-molecule inhibitor) that promotes cancer-cell division (mutated tyrosine-kinase enzyme). The drug is given by mouth and turns off the signal for cell division. With this treatment the blood count returns to normal and the spleen is no longer enlarged. The patient's response can be monitored by tests searching for the presence of the abnormal chromosome. This test (called a polymerase chain-reaction (PCR) test is looking for minute quantities of the abnormal DNA or genetic material responsible for the cancer-cell change.

An alternative treatment for younger patients who have a compatible donor is bone-marrow transplantation. This can cure some 60–70% of patients. However, it has severe side effects and requires several weeks in hospital.

In some patients a more acute and more dangerous form of this disease will develop, resembling acute myeloid leukaemia. This phase of the disease is more difficult to control. Cytotoxic chemotherapy with cortisone might give control for a period.

Chronic lymphocytic leukaemia

Chronic lymphocytic leukaemia tends to occur in older people of an average age of 60. In this disease there is an overproduction of mature and relatively normal-looking lymphocytes, with increased numbers of lymphocytes in the blood. (Lymphocytes are one of the main types of white cells in the blood. They are in high concentration in lymph nodes and some other tissues.)

Symptoms and signs

The most obvious feature of this cancer is lymph-node enlargement. Enlarged lymph nodes may be felt as lumps in the sides of the neck or in the armpits (axillae) or groins. Enlarged lymph nodes in the abdomen are more difficult to feel, but enlarged lymph nodes in the chest may be detected on a chest X-ray. The spleen and liver may also sometimes be enlarged. The normal bone marrow may be replaced by malignant lymphocytes, and the patient may become anaemic (deficient in red cells) and deficient in the circulating clotting particles called platelets. This may lead to bleeding and clotting problems. Due to the replacement of normal white cells by abnormal white cells, the patient has a decreased ability to combat infection and may also have immunologic abnormalities. Currently the majority of patients are actually diagnosed when asymptomatic (having no symptoms) after a blood count for some other reason. This asymptomatic state may last for many years.

Investigations

Blood count, a bone-marrow biopsy and special immune tests (tests of cell surface markers on the abnormal lymphocytes) will establish the diagnosis.

Treatment

Chronic lymphocytic leukaemia is usually a very slowly progressing disease, and many patients may not need treatment for many years. There is no evidence that the disease can be cured by early treatment, and treatment is usually reserved for episodes of the disease that are causing the patient to feel ill or causing other problems.

Large and conspicuous lymph nodes and a large spleen can be reduced by radiotherapy. If the patient's general health is poor, treatment with anti-cancer cytotoxic drugs, often with cortisone, will usually cause reduction of enlarged lymph nodes and spleen and improve the bone marrow, and will make the patient feel better. Two cytotoxic anti-cancer drugs are commonly used: chlorambucil and cyclophosphamide. Both are given by mouth. Newer active drugs include the antimetabolite fludarabine and the monoclonal antibody Mabthera.

Unlike chronic myeloid leukaemia, chronic lymphatic leukaemia does not degenerate into an acute type of leukaemia. However, it may occasionally change into a lymphoma-like disease, as described below.

The lymphomas

The lymphomas are a group of malignant diseases (cancers) of the tissues that constitute the body-defence system called the reticuloendothelial or immune system. That is, the lymphomas arise in lymph nodes or in lymphoid tissue elsewhere, such as the tonsils, the spleen, the wall of the stomach or bowel, the liver, lung, kidneys or skin.

There are two main types of lymphoma: Hodgkin lymphoma (previously called Hodgkin's disease) and the so-called non-Hodgkin lymphomas (NHL).

Currently about 12% of cases are Hodgkin lymphoma. The incidence of this disease has remained stable, while that of non-Hodgkin lymphoma has progressively increased over recent decades. The reasons for this are not clear.

Lymphomas are the sixth most common cause of death from cancer in Australia and commonly occur in young people. The average age is about 30 for Hodgkin lymphoma and a little over 40 for non-Hodgkin lymphoma.

The causes of most lymphomas are not known. Viruses are known to be a cause of lymphomas in some animals but, with one exception, they have not been found to be a significant cause of lymphoma in humans. A lymphoma called Burkitt's lymphoma, which is uncommon in most countries but is common in children in tropical Africa and New Guinea, has been found to be associated with infection by the Epstein-Barr virus. This same virus causes glandular fever, and it has been found that in Western societies people who have suffered from glandular fever have a slightly increased risk of developing a lymphoma later in life. On the other hand, doctors and nurses who specialise in caring for people with lymphoma have not been found to have any increased risk of developing the disease.

It is well recognised that people with a deficiency of the immune system, especially AIDS patients, but also others (such as people who have had a kidney transplant and are given drugs to suppress the rejection of the transplanted kidney), have an increased risk of developing a lymphoma. There is also a slightly increased tendency to develop lymphomas in some families, but this may be due to a hereditary tendency towards immune deficiency.

Hodgkin lymphoma
Symptoms and signs
The most common sign of this disease, especially in young people, is enlarged lymph nodes, usually in one side of the neck.

The nodes are rubbery and movable and usually feel distinctly different to the hard enlarged nodes that may result from secondary spread from other cancers.

Sometimes other symptoms are present: malaise (a general feeling of ill health), fever or weight loss. Occasionally pain in swollen lymph nodes following drinking alcohol is a feature.

The disease usually progresses from the site of origin (most commonly lymph nodes in the neck) to other lymph nodes nearby, then to lymph nodes in the chest or abdomen, to the spleen, and eventually to the liver and bone marrow. The earlier the disease is detected before it has spread widely, the greater the likelihood of cure by modern treatment.

Investigations

In order to decide on the best treatment for a patient it is important to find out as accurately as possible which lymph nodes and which organs are involved with this form of cancer. If this disease is suspected, the doctor performs a thorough examination of the patient, including all lymph-node areas, spleen, liver and chest. CT scans of the chest and abdomen can reveal enlarged lymph nodes, and this is complemented by PET scanning if it is available. Blood counts are also done, including tests relating to malignancy, such as the erythrocyte sedimentation reaction (ESR) and serum lactate dehydrogenase (serum LDH) tests.

The doctor then makes sure of the diagnosis by having the most obvious and easily removed lymph node excised by a surgeon and examined under a microscope. Any patient who has a non-tender lymph node greater than 2–3 cm in diameter remaining enlarged for more than four to six weeks without an obvious cause should have that node removed and examined. This will allow diagnosis or exclusion of lymphomas or other serious disease. In Asia or Africa tuberculosis sometimes mimics all the clinical features of lymphoma. Examination of excised lymph nodes will distinguish the diseases. A bone-marrow biopsy may be done in certain patients.

Treatment

Previously patients with Hodgkin lymphoma had an abdominal operation to determine how advanced the lymphoma was and what tissues were diseased. That operation involved removing some lymph nodes and often the spleen, and possibly a biopsy of the liver, all to be examined microscopically. It is now virtually never performed, due to the accuracy of CT and PET scanning.

Treatment of Hodgkin lymphoma depends on the stage of the disease and includes chemo/radiotherapy or chemotherapy alone. Treatment must be given by experts experienced in treating this disease, usually in multidisciplinary teams in specialised centres. It is now possible to cure the majority of patients.

In general limited areas of disease are best treated by an initial course of combination chemotherapy followed by radiotherapy to the areas of original disease. Modern linear accelerators are the most appropriate equipment for radiation therapy. The exact doses, techniques of delivery and field of irradiation are planned using sophisticated computer technology.

For more widespread disease treatment usually involves more extensive courses of combination chemotherapy. Again, to achieve best results and to keep toxicity to a minimum (see Section 2), treatment should be given by experts who are familiar with the use of these drugs and experienced in treating lymphomas. There have been considerable improvements in the chemotherapies available, with a reduction in immediate and long-term toxicity.

Non-Hodgkin lymphoma (NHL)

Like Hodgkin lymphoma, this group of diseases begins in reticuloendothelial or lymphatic tissues (the immune defence system) and is most commonly found in lymph nodes. However, the first indication of NHL may be the enlargement of, or lumps in, the spleen, tonsils or other organs such as the stomach, bowel, lung, bone or skin.

Non-Hodgkin lymphoma is not just one disease but a complex and wide range of diseases. The particular type of lymphoma depends upon the predominant type of malignant cells involved and their behaviour. The key issue is the type of lymphoma. They usually fall into three main classes according to their clinical behaviour or level of aggressiveness: low-grade, intermediate and high-grade forms.

Investigations

Diagnosis is usually made by surgical removal of an enlarged lymph node or biopsy of a lump in another tissue with microscopic examination.

Non-Hodgkin lymphomas tend to behave according to the predominant type of malignant cell. As with Hodgkin lymphoma, operations involving the removal and examination of potentially affected tissues are rarely needed. In the non-Hodgkin lymphomas the disease tends to involve a number of tissues other than lymph nodes, and the best form of treatment will depend upon the predominant type of malignant cell rather than the types of tissue involved. However, investigations similar to those for Hodgkin lymphoma are usually required. These include full blood count, CT scan of chest and abdomen, bone-marrow biopsy, liver biopsy and, increasingly, PET scans as they become more widely available (see Section 2).

Treatment

Just as for Hodgkin lymphoma, treatment of the non-Hodgkin lymphomas is by radiotherapy, chemotherapy or both. However, depending on the type of lymphoma, different plans of radiotherapy or different programs of chemotherapy are used. It is therefore essential that the patient be treated by a team of experts who can best determine the type and extent of disease and arrange the most appropriate plan of treatment.

In general, radiotherapy is best used for localised disease. With the non-Hodgkin lymphomas, however, there is a considerable risk that the disease is present in more than one site or in more than one tissue, and treatment by general body chemotherapy (systemic chemotherapy) is usually required. Sometimes the use of one cytotoxic agent only will achieve good results, but in general the best results are achieved when a combination of two or more cytotoxic drugs is used.

Over recent years the results of treatment of most non-Hodgkin lymphomas have improved significantly with modern treatment regimens. This is especially the case for some specific types of lymphoma. For some younger patients, even with advanced disease, very-high-dose toxic treatment followed by a bone-marrow transplant may be used with a good chance of success. A major improvement in treatment outcome has been the result of the development of a genetically engineered antibody directed against the lymphoma cells. This is produced using biotechnology industrial processes using mouse cells to produce a humanised antibody. The antibody is named Mabthera (ritiximab) and is used in combination with chemotherapy. The results of treatment for some of the early-stage lymphomas can be excellent, with a high cure rate, particularly for the so-called diffuse large B cell lymphomas.

SOFT-TISSUE SARCOMAS

The soft tissues are those that surround the bones of the body. They include muscles, fat, fascia, nerves, tendons, blood vessels and lymphatic vessels. A malignant tumour of one of these tissues is a 'sarcoma'. However, the general term 'cancer' is often used to include sarcomas as they are a malignancy in many ways similar to cancer.

The majority of soft-tissue tumours are not malignant; it is only when they are malignant that the term sarcoma applies. Most tumours of fatty tissue are lipomas; when one of these is malignant, it is called a liposarcoma. Similarly, most tumours of fibrous tissue are benign and are called fibromas, and most tumours of nerves are benign and are called neuromas. Most blood- and lymph-vessel tumours are benign and are called angiomas.

Thus, sarcomas are classified according to the type of tissue from which they arise and the type of tissue they most resemble. A fibrosarcoma is a malignant tumour or cancer of fibrous tissue; a liposarcoma is a malignant tumour or cancer of fatty tissue; a neurofibrosarcoma is a malignant tumour or cancer of nerve tissue; a malignant fibrous histiocytoma (MFH) is a sarcoma of histiocytes (the protective cells most often found in soft tissues); and a synovial sarcoma is a malignant tumour of the synovial membrane that lines joints and tendon sheaths.

A myosarcoma is a malignant tumour of muscle. Myosarcomas may be further classified as rhabdomyosarcoma or leiomyosarcoma. A rhabdomyosarcoma is a malignant tumour of a voluntary muscle (that is, one of the muscles of the body over which we have movement control, such as those in our arms, legs, abdomen, back, head and neck, and the muscles used in breathing). A leiomyosarcoma is a malignant tumour of involuntary muscle (that is, one of the muscles over which we have no conscious control, such as the muscle in the wall of the stomach or bowel, and the muscles in the wall of the uterus or the wall of large blood vessels).

An angiosarcoma is a malignant tumour of blood or lymph vessels. In the case of blood vessels it is called a haemangiosarcoma, or in the case of lymphatic vessels it is called lymphangiosarcoma.

Soft-tissue sarcomas occur in people of all ages from birth to old age, but they are much less common than true cancers. Soft-tissue sarcomas make up only about 2% of malignant tumours.

In general sarcomas have a tendency to recur locally after surgical excision and also to spread. While most cancers tend to spread via the lymph vessels to lymph nodes before they spread to lungs or other body organs, most sarcomas tend to spread via blood vessels to lungs rather than to lymph nodes.

Classification-pathological types
Fibrosarcoma
Fibrosarcomas develop in the fascia or fibrous tissue that covers and surrounds muscles, nerves and other tissues and is distributed widely throughout the body. Thus a fibrosarcoma may develop almost anywhere in the body, especially in a limb or in the tissues of the trunk. One very fibrous and slow-growing type of fibrosarcoma, called a desmoid tumour, has a tendency to grow into nearby tissues and to recur locally after surgical

excision but rarely spreads to other organs. Other more cellular and less fibrous types have a greater tendency to spread.

Liposarcoma

These tumours develop from fatty tissue and may arise anywhere in the body where fat is present. They tend to vary from a low-grade malignancy likely to recur locally after removal but unlikely to spread to a high-grade malignancy in which both local recurrence and secondary spread to lungs is common.

Rhabdomyosarcoma

This malignant tumour presents as a swelling in voluntary muscle, especially in muscles in the limbs, and is the sarcoma most likely to spread to lymph nodes.

Leiomyosarcoma

This malignant tumour may occur at any site where there is smooth muscle, including the wall of the stomach, bowel or uterus, or the wall of large blood vessels.

Neurofibrosarcoma

This malignant tumour may develop in any nerve. Tumours of the nerve sheath are termed 'malignant peripheral nerve sheath tumours', while those originating in the actual nerve fibre may be termed 'primitive neuroectodermal tumours' or 'neuroblastomas' or 'ganglioneuroblastomas'.

Malignant fibrous histiocytoma (MFH)

These tumours most commonly develop in muscles, fascia or fatty tissues in limbs. They are firm, rounded tumours rather like liposarcomas or fibrosarcomas. If they are sited deep in the muscle, they may become quite large before they are noticed as they cause few symptoms until a lump is felt.

Angiosarcoma

These malignant tumours may develop in relation to blood vessels or lymph vessels as enlarging vascular masses (clumps containing partly formed blood vessels). They are softish tumours that may contain either blood or lymphatic fluid. Prior to effective antiviral therapy an unusual form of blood-vessel tumour was seen in the skin and gastrointestinal tract of patients with AIDS, called Kaposi's sarcoma. It is very rare today but is occasionally seen in elderly males of Mediterranean ethnicity.

Synovial sarcoma (synovio sarcoma or malignant synovioma)

This tumour of the synovial membrane is often highly aggressive and malignant, and occurs most commonly in limbs near joints or in association with the sheaths around muscle tendons.

Symptoms and signs

Sarcomas occasionally develop from previously benign tumours of a similar type. Occasionally a previously benign lipoma, for example, will begin to enlarge, showing evidence of a malignant liposarcoma. More often, however, these cancers arise as a local swelling from no apparent pre-existing abnormality. Usually the lump is not painful, although sometimes there is some pain. Occasionally the swelling develops at a site of recent injury. It is more likely, however, that in most cases the injury drew attention to a lump that was already present.

Rarely the first evidence of a soft-tissue sarcoma is found in a chest X-ray showing as secondary lung cancer.

Investigations

The examining doctor will first ask about the lump, especially how long it has been present and if, when and how rapidly it started to enlarge. The lump is measured, the local draining lymph nodes and other lymph nodes examined and a chest X-ray and full blood count performed. An MRI scan, ultrasound and angiography (see Section 2) may also give more information about the tumour, particularly the degree of invasion or compression of surrounding tissues. MRI scans provide more information in this regard than CT scans. The definitive diagnosis is made by a biopsy of the tumour for microscopic examination. The role of PET scanning is still being investigated.

Treatment

The standard treatment of soft-tissue sarcoma is surgical excision. As the risk of local recurrence is high, the surgeon must remove a great deal of apparently normal tissue around the tumour to be as sure as possible that all of the malignant cells have been removed. In some circumstances large tumours in a limb may require amputation. This can sometimes be avoided by using induction (neoadjuvant) chemotherapy or chemo/radiotherapy to shrink the tumour prior to surgery.

In some specialised clinics the chemotherapy can be given by regional infusion into a supplying artery (as in the case of sarcoma in a limb), with good responses in shrinking the cancer. Amputation has been avoided in 80% of patients who would have previously been treated this way. Similar responses are seen if the chemotherapy is given over an hour or so in a 'closed circuit infusion', and even better responses have been reported when the immunologic agent TNF is included in the closed circuit.

Although these cancers are usually not particularly sensitive to radiotherapy, chemo/radiotherapy followed by local surgery may allow resection of large cancers, especially in the head, thorax, abdomen or pelvis. Liposarcomas and malignant fibrous histiocytomas are the most common of the soft-tissue sarcomas encountered in this way.

With some sarcomas the risk of secondary spread to the lungs is considerable, and there may be virtue in also giving a post-operative course of adjuvant chemotherapy (see Section 2) to reduce this risk. It appears this may only be of value, however, when the primary sarcoma is located on a limb. In some patients isolated metastases such as those in the lung may be surgically excised.

MALIGNANT TUMOURS OF BONE AND CARTILAGE

Osteosarcoma

A malignant tumour of bone-forming cells is called an osteo-sarcoma. This is an uncommon but highly malignant form of cancer and tends to affect children and young adults, with the highest incidence between ten and 25 years of age. The cause of osteosarcoma in young people is not known, although it does occur most often in the growth plates (the growing centres) near the bone ends while the patient is still growing.

A rare and incurable osteosarcoma sometimes develops in old people in the site of a chronic bone disease called osteitis deformans (Paget's disease of bone).

Symptoms and signs

Osteosarcoma usually first develops as a painful swelling near the end of a bone in a child or young adult. This may be associated with overlying redness and sometimes a fever. The swelling may be tender and may at first look like an acute infection in the bone. This sarcoma tends to spread to the lungs early in its course, so best results are achieved if it is diagnosed and treated as soon as possible.

Investigations

Bone X-rays often show a typical appearance of the disease from which a preliminary diagnosis of osteosarcoma can be made.

More precise information can be learned from CT studies or MRI studies. PET scanning is still under investigation. However, diagnosis depends on a bone biopsy in which a small piece of the tumour is taken for microscopic examination. Chest CT scans are carried out to look for metastases in the lungs.

Treatment

Prior to the development of effective adjuvant chemotherapy osteosarcoma was fatal in the majority of patients. Treatment was by early amputation of an affected limb, sometimes in combination with radiotherapy, but death usually resulted due to the development of secondary cancer in the lungs.

The outlook has been greatly improved with modern chemotherapy. Nowadays cytotoxic drugs are given as induction (or neoadjuvant) chemotherapy (see Section 2) from the time of diagnosis up to surgery. Not long ago amputation was usually used to remove the primary sarcoma followed by chemotherapy to eradicate any microscopic secondary cancers in the lungs. From a 20% cure rate improvement in survival has increased to over 50%. A further advance has been limb conservation. Instead of amputation, after chemotherapy it is possible in many patients to locally resect the remaining cancer mass. An internal prosthesis made of special metal or plastic is then used to reconstruct the limb. In some specialised centres the induction chemotherapy is given via a cannula inserted into the artery directly supplying the tumour. This combined treatment is very effective in curing more than half of the patients with osteosarcoma, and in 80% of these cases the cure is achieved without amputating the limb.

In some clinics the pre-operative chemotherapy is not given into the artery supplying the limb but is given systemically (into a vein). This is an easier method of giving chemotherapy, and the results of treatment are possibly as good as with intra-arterial chemotherapy for this cancer.

Osteoclastoma (central giant cell tumour of bone)

This cancer occurs most commonly in the ends of the long bones of middle-aged adults. It is a cancer of low-grade malignancy, in that it does not often spread to other organs or tissues but tends to develop locally and commonly recurs locally after attempts at removal.

Symptoms and signs

The first evidence of this tumour is usually swelling, often with pain. It may be first noticed due to a fracture of the weakened bone.

Investigations

X-rays or CT or MRI scans will usually show a typical appearance of this tumour, but diagnosis is established by the surgeon taking a biopsy specimen and having it examined by a pathologist under the microscope.

Treatment

If possible, the tumour is removed surgically. If it is inadequately removed, radiotherapy may be given post-operatively.

A recurrent tumour tends to be more malignant, however, and treatment by amputation may be required.

Ewing's tumour

This is an uncommon malignant tumour that occurs most often in the shafts of the long bones of adolescents and young adults between the age of ten and the late teenage years. Although it occurs in bones, it is not truly a tumour of bone cells but a tumour of connective tissue in bone.

Symptoms and signs

Pain, swelling, fever and anaemia are common features of Ewing's tumour, so much so that a diagnosis of infection (osteomyelitis) may be considered. Sometimes lesions are present in more than one bone.

Investigations

X-rays of the bone often show the laminated 'onion peel' appearance that is typical of Ewing's tumour. Further useful information may be gained from CT or MRI studies or from isotope scans. Biopsy and microscopic examination will establish the diagnosis.

This is a tumour where, if available, PET scans may be

especially helpful to detect any centres of malignant growth in bones at other sites and to see evidence of a response to chemotherapy and radiotherapy treatment.

Treatment

Standard treatment by surgery (usually amputation) has rarely cured this highly malignant tumour. Adjuvant chemotherapy is critical in preventing metastatic disease.

With modern treatment using chemotherapy, radiotherapy and possibly local surgical excision significantly better results are now being achieved.

Multiple myeloma

This is a malignant tumour of plasma cells, occurring in the bone marrow. Normal plasma cells are derived from lymphocytes, and their role is to produce antibodies in response to infection or vaccination. The malignant plasma cells often produce a single type of antibody-like protein molecule. This is called a paraprotein and can be measured in the blood by special electophoretic tests. The abnormal plasma cells may be scattered through the bone marrow, crowding out the normal (haemopoeitic) marrow that produces red cells, white cells and platelets. This may cause the patient to become anaemic and at risk of infection or bleeding. In some patients the paraprotein may damage the kidneys. Also the plasma cells may form a large number of tumours growing inside bones. These can cause so-called lytic lesions or areas where bone has been dissolved away, resulting in severe pain or even fracture of major bones. If a patient has only one such lesion, this is called a plasmacytoma.

Multiple myeloma most often affects adults over the age of 50, and its cause in most patients is not known. However, radiation exposure is a risk factor, and the disease, for unknown reasons, is more common in African Americans.

Investigations

X-rays may show typical 'punched out' or lytic areas in bones. A blood count is taken, as the patients are usually found to have anaemia. The presence of a paraprotein, together with a bone-marrow biopsy, will confirm the diagnosis.

The urine is also examined for a segment of the paraprotein (Bence-Jones protein), which, if present, indicates a diagnosis of multiple myeloma. This protein is also a risk factor for kidney damage.

Treatment

Solitary plasmacytomas are surgically removed, followed by local radiation therapy. Younger patients (i.e. those less than 65–70 years old) can be treated with high-dose chemotherapy and haemopoietic cell support with a cytokine called granulocyte colony-stimulating factor (G CSF) to build up the blood. This can result in disease remission and survival for several years in some patients. This therapy is relatively toxic, however, and requires some weeks in hospital. For older or frailer patients treatment with simpler forms of therapy, including intermittent courses of high-dose cortisone drugs, can be effective. Thalidomide has also been shown to be of value in this disease. It appears to inhibit small-blood-vessel formation in the marrow, thus inhibiting growth of the abnormal plasma cells.

Chondrosarcoma

Chondrosarcoma is a malignant tumour of cartilage and most often affects middle-aged adults. This tumour may develop on any bone, especially at the ends of long bones or in the bones of the pelvis. It is usually first noticed as a slow-growing painful lump on a bone, often near a large joint.

Investigations

X-rays will often show the typical appearance of a chondrosarcoma, but a biopsy is required to establish the diagnosis. CT or MRI studies will help show the exact position, nature and extent of the tumour.

Treatment

If possible, radical surgical excision of the tumour and adjacent bone is carried out. This may require amputation of a limb.

These sarcomas are not sensitive to standard radiotherapy or to chemotherapy, but as they are slow growing and usually do not spread until late in the disease, treatment by radical surgery usually results in cure.

METASTATIC (SECONDARY) CANCER

A secondary or metastatic cancer is a cancer that is growing in an organ or tissue some distance away from the tissue or organ in which it originated. Benign tumours tend to grow very slowly and remain localised to the tissues in which they arise, whereas malignant tumours (cancers) tend to grow more rapidly, to grow into surrounding structures and damage them, and to spread into tissues or organs away from the original or primary site of development.

To spread to distant sites, the malignant cells usually grow into blood vessels or lymph vessels, and clumps of cells break off and are carried by the bloodstream or the lymphatic vessels to a distant organ or tissue, or to lymph nodes, where they may grow as secondary tumours. The spreading cancer cells can be thought of as 'seeds' being transported along blood or lymph vessels to a new 'soil', where they may take root and grow. Malignant cells may also sometimes spread along nerve sheaths, or across body cavities such as the abdominal cavity or a pleural cavity in the chest.

The most common site for the secondary spread of cancers is via lymph vessels into lymph nodes. First they grow in lymph nodes near the original cancer and then spread into lymph nodes further away. The next most common sites are the lungs or the liver, which they access through the bloodstream.

Other common sites of secondary spread are to bones, under the skin or to the ovaries. No tissue is exempt from developing a secondary cancer. This includes the thyroid, adrenal and other glands, the bowel, brain, spinal cord, limbs, testes, uterus, skin, bladder or kidneys. It should be noted, though, that some organs and tissues tend to have a relatively low incidence of secondary growth of most cancers for no obvious reason. These include the spleen and muscles.

The likelihood of a tumour spreading to a particular site depends very much on the type of tumour and its place of origin. Stomach, pancreas and bowel cancers, for example, tend to spread first to abdominal lymph nodes and to the liver. Breast cancer tends to spread to nearby lymph nodes, usually first to nodes in the armpit and then to more distant lymph nodes, to the liver, lungs and bone. Prostate cancer tends to spread to nearby lymph nodes and to bone. Skin cancer and cancers in the mouth and throat tend to spread to nearby lymph nodes; the exception is BCC, which rarely spreads anywhere other than into surrounding tissues. Melanoma, on the other hand, tends to spread early not only to lymph nodes but to almost any other organ or tissue in the body.

Sarcomas do not usually spread to lymph nodes first: they are more likely to first spread via the bloodstream to the lungs.

More detail about the spread of each different type of cancer has been discussed under the relevant headings earlier in this section. The treatment of secondary cancer depends on the type and site of origin of the particular cancer; treatment has similarly been discussed under the individual headings in this section.

4

where do we go from here?

THE FUTURE

The future for cancer patients should be viewed with a mixture of hope and caution. Certainly there is much that can be done to treat cancers through the skilled application of present knowledge. There is also great reason to expect improvements in prevention, diagnosis and care in the future.

However, just as there will be great advances in the prevention and management of cancer in the future, so too will there be new challenges. The condition AIDS is one such example: it is a new health problem unknown 35 years ago. Affected people have increased susceptibility to infections and to malignant tumour development, especially lymphoma or Kaposi's sarcoma. The discovery of new antiviral drugs has led to control of the disease manifestations in patients with AIDS but not a cure. These patients now live a relatively normal life without the severe infections or malignancy.

People who have had organ transplants and are dependent on immunosuppressive drugs to prevent rejection of the organ also have an increased risk of developing cancer. This also is a relatively new problem, unknown 40 years ago.

The sexual revolution has exposed young women to an increased risk of cancer of the cervix. However, there is an expectation that the new vaccine available will, in the future, eliminate cervical cancer just as polio was eliminated.

It is not known what potential other modern drugs, especially illegal drugs, might have to increase the risk of cancer. It was many years before the dangers of tobacco smoking became obvious. Studies suggest that for long-term smokers of marijuana, the risk of cancer is similar to that for tobacco smokers.

PREVENTION

The most obvious way to reduce the risk of cancer is to avoid smoking. This has been known for some years but, human nature being what it is, this precaution has been widely disregarded. As long as there are large profits to be made from the sale of tobacco products, there will be resistance to the introduction of statutory measures aimed at reducing smoking.

Another useful measure is to encourage fair-skinned people to take greater protection against exposure to the sun.

More attention can also be paid to removal of pre-malignant

conditions such as hyperkeratoses, leukoplakia, stomach and bowel polyps and papillomas, and to the prevention of such infections as hepatitis and HIV.

Diet and changes in lifestyle

Changes in lifestyle should include a reduction of animal fats, artificial additives and other contaminants in the diet, and a greater intake of fibre, fresh fish, fresh fruits and vegetables, nuts and protective legumes. This sensible diet will also reduce the risks of obesity, diabetes and cardiovascular disease. Moderation in the use of alcohol should be encouraged.

There will continue to be advances in understanding of the role of diet based on epidemiological information and a better understanding of the protective qualities of high-fibre diets, and of the apparent protective qualities of other agents, such as the naturally occurring hormones (phytoestrogens) present in soy and other plant foods and the antioxidants such as lycopene, the red colouring matter in tomatoes and some other red fruits.

Open-mindedness towards 'alternative' and naturopathic practices

More might be learned from alternative medicine and naturo-pathic practices as well as traditional practices from ancient and undeveloped communities. Several effective anti-cancer drugs are extracted from plants used in other cultures, and it is likely that other such anti-cancer agents will be discovered among plants being used in other cultures or by alternative practices. However, care must be taken to properly analyse such practices and not allow wishful thinking, emotion or fashion to cloud scientific and clinical judgement.

Improved environmental and industrial laws and practices

The reduction of atmospheric pollutants, vigilant observation of protective industrial laws and protection against radioactive sources are other important factors in the prevention of cancer.

Improved cancer screening

Another measure of increasing importance is regular screening of people at special risk for certain types of cancer so that any early lesions can be detected and treated before an advanced cancer develops. At present this seems to be the most appropriate way to detect early breast cancer, skin cancers including melanoma, cancer of the cervix, cancer of the stomach (in some countries) and large-bowel cancer.

It is anticipated that simpler and more accurate screening measures will be available in the future. These may involve simple blood-screening tests for cancer antibodies or other tumour markers to indicate the presence of cancer before symptoms have developed and at a more curable stage. The recognition that heredity plays a role in certain families, together with predictive DNA testing, will also play a larger role in the future.

EARLY DETECTION AND TREATMENT: IMPROVED DIAGNOSTIC TECHNIQUES

Improved diagnostic measures will also allow more accurate diagnosis at an earlier stage. Already, improvements in CT scanning and other organ-imaging techniques have made considerable advances, and further advances are assured. Magnetic resonance imaging (MRI) has added to these improved diagnostic and imaging methods. It is anticipated that the newer method of organ imaging, PET (positron emission tomography), may make an even greater impact within a few years because of the additional information it gives about the activity, composition and survival of tumour cells and its capacity to detect secondary cells at an earlier stage than has been possible in the past.

Fine-needle aspiration cytology, frozen-section techniques and other improved pathology techniques have allowed major progress in detecting and establishing the nature of tumours. Improvements in the ability to examine body cavities with the use of flexible fibrescopes have allowed considerable progress in detecting and assessing early cancers in recent years, too. These instruments and their applications will undoubtedly continue to be improved.

IMPROVED AGENTS AND MORE EFFECTIVE USE OF CHEMOTHERAPY

Improvements in treatment, with more effective and more specific anti-cancer drugs, is ongoing. So too is knowledge of how best to use such drugs in combinations and appropriate treatment schedules for achieving greater anti-tumour effects with a reduced risk of toxicity and unwanted side effects. New and more effective anti-cancer agents such as monoclonal antibodies or small designer drugs directed at specific cancer-cell targets are now producing, in combination with chemotherapy, improved outcomes for a wide range of cancers. Many drugs are being made safer and more effective with the increasing availability of agents that protect bone marrow and other body tissues.

Advances in molecular biology coupled with the sequencing of the human genome have led to analysis of the arrangement of DNA in genes in a genome (called microarray) of common human cancers. This is leading to a more accurate prediction of long-term outcomes and better selection of treatment modalities for individual patients in various clinical trials.

IMPROVEMENTS IN RADIOTHERAPY

Treatment by radiotherapy is also being constantly improved, with sophisticated computer-planning technology coupled with CT, MRI and PET scans that accurately image tumour targets. The ability to combine radiotherapy with chemotherapy has improved treatment results too. More effective use of chemotherapy and radiotherapy integrated with surgery can be anticipated as cancer specialists become better organised in multidisciplinary teams focusing on specific cancer types. The best example of this has been in the treatment of breast cancer. The combined effects of earlier diagnosis with less mutilating surgery and either adjuvant chemotherapy or hormonal therapy has seen the death rate from this disease fall by over 20% in the last 15 years.

Newer forms of radiation therapy are available and being tested in trials in a small number of world specialist centres. One such form is a Cyberknife, which is basically an advanced linear-accelerator technique that rotates around the cancer region, focusing the irradiation onto a limited central region. This equipment and technique is being especially studied in Washington DC. Another newly developed treatment is proton-beam therapy, which directs irradiation to deep, specially targeted cancers. This equipment and technique is being chiefly studied in Boston and in Loma Linda in California. Another recent development in radiotherapy is the use of a neutron beam. Early studies show it to be effective in treating an otherwise resistant type of salivary-gland tumour called an adenocystic carcinoma.

HEAT THERAPY AND CRYOSURGERY

Another treatment possibility, as yet not well exploited, involves the known increased susceptibility of cancer cells to heat. Studies of the application of heat to selectively eradicate cancer cells, possibly in combination with anti-cancer drugs, may produce improved treatment techniques for certain types of cancer in the future. At the same time the application of extreme cold to cancer cells (cryosurgery) is being further developed, especially as a technique to cure secondary cancers in the liver.

IMMUNOTHERAPY

An enormous amount of research in universities, hospitals and cancer-research institutions is attempting to better understand the role of immunological defence mechanisms against cancer. There is hope that specific immunological tumour markers will lead to earlier diagnosis of certain cancers. This would improve outcomes, for instance, in ovarian cancer. Monoclonal tumour antibodies are now widely used in the treatment of certain forms of breast cancer and lymphoma, and their use may extend to many other tumour types. There is hope that a more reliable means of stimulating the immune defence system through various vaccine-like treatments may also emerge, despite many negative past results. Studies with products of the immune defence system such as interferon and the interleukins (see Section 2) have not as yet had the impact originally expected.

GENETIC ENGINEERING

New techniques of molecular DNA biology offer a different approach to combating cancer. It may soon be possible to change the structure of DNA in cells and thus change the nature of actually or potentially malignant cells into cells without the properties of malignant growth. The new science of genetic engineering also has potential for changing the basic nature of cells to prevent cancer developing or to change the nature of malignant cells.

TARGETED SMALL-MOLECULE SIGNAL INHIBITORS

There is now a very detailed understanding of the growth and cell division of biochemical pathways in normal and cancer cells. Specific mutations or changes in these pathways are responsible for the abnormal growth of cancer cells. Many new drugs have been and continue to be developed that specifically inhibit these steps. (The best known is a drug called Glivec, which is very effective in treating chronic myeloid leukaemia.) These are being introduced into clinical trials in conjunction with the older chemotherapy drugs, with improved outcomes in several cancer types.

IMPROVED PALLIATIVE CARE

For those people with advanced cancer and in great discomfort or pain, methods of relieving the suffering are now better understood. Such measures are now more readily available and there is little need for patients to suffer greatly from pain or other distressing symptoms of cancer. These facilities will be further improved and made more readily available to those who need them.

HOPE FOR THE FUTURE

For those with serious but not terminal disease, there are now good prospects for recovery: there is a probability of cure for increasing numbers of patients with cancer. Today, even excluding the relatively simple skin cancers, overall cure rates are well over 50%. Even for those with what is still considered to be terminal disease, worthwhile palliation is available to improve quality of life, and there remains the hope that for some, further improvement in treatment methods may soon bring a better prospect of cure.

glossary

ACUTE Having a sudden, severe and short course.

ADENOCARCINOMA A malignant tumour (cancer) that began in gland cells or glandular cells lining a body cavity.

ADENOMA A benign (not malignant) tumour in which the cells are derived from glands or from glandular epithelium such as the lining of the stomach.

ANAEMIA A blood condition with reduced numbers of red blood cells and/or a reduced amount of haemoglobin.

> **Pernicious anaemia** A type of anaemia resulting from a failure of gastric mucosa (stomach lining) to produce a vital ingredient for making blood called 'intrinsic factor'.

ANALOGUE A drug that differs in minor ways from its original compound.

ANOREXIA A feeling of not wanting to eat (lack of hunger).

ANTIBODY A particle manufactured in the immune system to defend the body against a harmful invading organism or particle called an antigen.

ARTERIOGRAM A radiograph (X-ray photograph) of an artery taken after injection of a radio-opaque substance (dye) into the artery.

ASBESTOS A fibrous silicate material that was mined for use in building and other industries. It is now known to be dangerous and if inhaled can cause mesothelioma or lung cancer.

ASPIRATION The act of sucking up or sucking out.

ASTROCYTOMA A malignant tumour of connective tissue cells in the brain.

ATROPHIC Wasted. Degenerate. Showing a loss of special qualities.

AXILLA Armpit.

BACTERIA Germs.

BARIUM *Barium meal* A chalky, porridge-like substance containing the radio-opaque element barium, which is swallowed to allow radiographs to be taken that enable the outline, size and shape of organs such as the stomach or duodenum to be seen on X-ray films or on an X-ray screen.

> **Barium swallow** Similar to a barium meal except that as the material is swallowed, X-ray films and screening of the oesophagus allow the shape and outline of the oesophagus to be studied.

> **Barium enema** Similar to a barium meal except the material is passed via a tube through the anus to allow X-ray films and screening of the rectum and large bowel.

BASAL Basic. The lowest or foundation part of a structure. The basal layer of skin cells consists of the deeper cells from which the surface cells grow.

BCC Basal-cell carcinoma. A slow-growing skin cancer that grows from the deep (basal) layer of skin cells.

BCG Bacille Calmette-Guérin. A preparation originally used as an active immunising agent against tuberculosis. It consists of harmless living organisms that promote a similar body-defence action to that of tuberculosis bacteria.

BENIGN Not malignant. Favourable for recovery. Unlikely to be dangerous.

BENIGN MAMMARY DYSPLASIA A condition of the breasts that is likely to cause cysts and other benign lumps in the breasts.

BIOPSY The removal of a small sample of body tissue for microscopic examination.

BUCCAL MUCOSA The lining of the cheek in the mouth.

CANCER A malignant, continuous, purposeless, unwanted and uncontrolled growth of cells.

CAPSULE The fibrous or membranous sac-like covering that encloses a tissue or an organ.

CARCINOGEN A substance that causes cancer.

CERVIX UTERI The neck of the uterus. The entrance of the womb.

CHEMOTHERAPY Treatment with chemical agents or drugs.

CHRONIC Persisting for a long time. Having a long or protracted course.

CHRONIC ATROPHIC GASTRITIS A gradual and persistent degeneration of the lining of the stomach.

CISPLATINUM A commonly used anti-cancer agent derived from the metal platinum. It binds DNA in cancer cells, causing DNA breaks and cell death. It is effective in treating a broad range of cancers, including breast, lung and head and neck cancers, especially when used in combination with other anti-cancer agents. Likely to cause nausea and vomiting, and can cause kidney damage if not used judiciously.

CONGENITAL Present from the time of birth.

CORTISONE A naturally occurring steroid hormone secreted by the adrenal gland.

CORYNEBACTERIUM PARVUM A harmless bacterium sometimes used to stimulate immune body-defence reactions.

CROHN'S DISEASE This name applies to granular colitis, an infection affecting the large bowel, and to a similar inflammatory condition that may affect the small intestine. The condition was first described by Dr Crohn.

CT (COMPUTERISED TOMOGRAPHY) SCAN A method of visualising body tissues by using special computerised radiographic techniques to give X-ray 'pictures' of sections of body tissues.

CYBERKNIFE A new form of radiotherapy that is basically an advanced linear accelarator that rotates around a tumour region focusing the irradiation onto a limited area containing the tumour.

CYTOKINES Protein materials released from cells when activated by antigens. Cytokines are involved in cell-to-cell communication enhancing immune reactions through specific cell-surface responses on white cells.

CYTOTOXIC Having a toxic or harmful effect upon cells.

DEXAMETHASONE A corticosteroid used mainly in treating allergic reactions.

DNA Deoxyribonucleic acid. The material from which the body-building genes and chromosomes are made.

ENDOSCOPE An instrument used for visual examination of the interior of hollow organs or the interior of body cavities.

EPIDEMIOLOGY The branch of medicine dealing with the distribution, incidence, causes and spread of diseases.

EPITHELIUM Tissue that forms a body-surface lining, such as a skin surface or the lining of a hollow organ that opens onto a body surface such as the lining of the mouth, bladder, bowel or vagina.

FAECES Stool.

FAMILIAL POLYPOSIS COLI An inherited condition in which about half of the members of a family will develop polyps (small tumours) in the wall of the large bowel. Eventually one or more of these will become malignant.

FASCIA *Superficial fascia* The fatty layer under the skin.

> **Fascia or deep fascia** The fibrous or membranous layer of tissue that covers muscles, nerves and blood vessels, or separates muscles or other tissues into different compartments.

FIBROMA A benign tumour composed of fibrous tissues and fibrous tissue-forming cells.

FLOOR OF MOUTH The lower part of the mouth under the tongue.

GASTROSCOPE An instrument used for visual examination of the interior of the stomach.

GENOME The total genetic material in an organism, comprising the genes contained in its chromosomes.

GLAND A tissue or organ that manufactures and secretes chemical substances necessary for the maintenance of normal health and body function.

GLUCAN A complex carbohydrate (type of sugar) that constitutes much of the fibre in common vegetable and grain foodstuffs, which has been found to have immune stimulatory properties.

GOITRE Enlargement of the thyroid gland causing a swelling in the front part of the neck.

GRANULOCYTE COLONY-STIMULATING FACTOR (G CSF) A growth factor or cytokine produced by tissues to stimulate the bone-marrow granuloctyes and stem cells.

HERCEPTIN A brand of human monoclonal antibody derived from DNA. It selectively targets cells with a certain human growth-factor protein on the cell surface.

HRT (HORMONE-REPLACEMENT THERAPY) Treatment with a low dose of hormones to reduce menopausal and post-menopausal symptoms and other problems such as loss of calcium from bones.

HYPERKERATOSIS A thickening of the flat protective surface layer of the epithelium of skin or lip. The condition is usually characterised by the formation of a crust or flakes that drop off. There can be a tendency for malignant changes to appear gradually, and cancer may develop.

IMMUNOTHERAPY The treatment of disease by giving immune substances or by stimulating the immune system of body defences.

INDURATION The hardening or thickening of a tissue or a part of the body as a local reaction due to inflammation or infiltration with cancer cells.

KAPOSI'S SARCOMA A malignant tumour that has developed in the blood vessels in skin. It appears as dark purple patches or nodules.

LESION An area of abnormal tissue with impaired function due to disease or injury.

LEUCOCYTE White cell. The 'white' or colourless type of cell that circulates in the blood, has amoeboid movement and is chiefly concerned with defending the body against invasion of foreign organisms or bacteria.

LEUKOPLAKIA White patch. A disease distinguished by the presence of white thickened patches in the mucous membranes, commonly in the mouth. There may be a tendency for malignant characteristics to appear gradually and thus for a cancer to develop.

LH-RH Luteinising hormone and releasing hormone. These are hormones released from the pituitary gland that stimulate other hormones, some of which may stimulate some cancers.

LIPOMA A benign tumour composed of fat cells.

LIVER The largest solid organ in the body. It lies in the upper abdomen predominantly on the right side and under cover of the lower-right ribs.

LYMPH NODES Small masses of lymphatic tissue 1–15 mm in diameter and normally bean-shaped. Scattered along the course of lymph vessels and often grouped in clusters, they form an important part of the body's defence system, functioning as factories for the development of lymphocytes and filtering bacteria and foreign debris from tissue fluid. They are sometimes referred to as 'lymph glands'.

LYMPH VESSELS or **LYMPHATICS** The small vessels that drain tissue fluid into lymph nodes and interconnect groups of lymph nodes. Eventually the larger lymph vessels drain this fluid into the bloodstream.

LYMPHANGIOGRAM A radiograph (X-ray photograph) of lymphatic vessels shown after they have been injected with a radio-opaque substance (dye).

LYMPHOCYTE One of the types of white cells that circulate in the blood and take part in immune reactions and the body's defence reactions. A mononuclear non-granular leucocyte produced by lymph nodes and other lymphoid tissue.

LYMPHOID Resembling or pertaining to the tissue of the lymphatic system. This tissue contains large numbers of round cells and produces lymphocytes.

LYMPHOMA A malignant tumour or cancer of lymphoid tissue.

MABTHERA A genetically engineered monoclonal antibody directed against a particular antigen on the cell surface of normal and malignant lymphocytes.

MALAISE A general feeling of lassitude and ill-health.

MALIGNANT Life-threatening. A condition which in the natural course of events would become progressively worse, resulting in death. A malignant growth or cancer is a growth of unwanted cells that tends to continue growing and invade, thus destroying surrounding tissues. It also tends to spread to other parts of the body, destroying other tissues.

MALIGNANT FIBROUS HISTIOCYTOMA A malignant tumour of histiocytes, which are protective (immune) cells in soft tissues (muscles, fat, etc.) or in bone.

MARJOLIN'S CANCER A cancer that has developed in a longstanding chronic ulcer.

MEDIASTINUM The central midline area of the chest. That part of the chest between the sternum (breast bone) and the vertebrae (back bone) containing the heart, great blood vessels, trachea and oesophagus.

MEDULLOBLASTOMA An uncommon malignant tumour that usually develops from primitive brain cells in the cerebellar part of the brain, most commonly in children and young people.

MELANOMA A malignant growth (cancer) of pigment-producing cells, most commonly arising in the skin, sometimes in the eye and occasionally elsewhere.

METASTASIS A secondary cancer that is growing in a tissue somewhere away from where it originally developed.

METASTATIC Metastatic cancer is a secondary growth of malignant cells that has spread from a primary cancer elsewhere.

MONOCLONAL An adjective that describes a particle of one special type only. A monoclonal antibody will affect one special chemical particle only and therefore the special type of cell that carries this particle.

MRI Magnetic resonance imaging. MRI scans allow X-ray-like pictures to be taken of cross-sections of the body, head or limbs. The resulting pictures are rather like those of CT scans.

MUCOUS MEMBRANE The lining of most hollow organs and some body cavities such as the mouth, stomach and bowel, all of which contain mucous glands and secrete mucus onto the surface.

MUCUS A protective slimy material secreted by certain glands and certain cells lining body cavities and hollow organs.

MUTATION A change in genetic material that causes a change in cell growth or activity.

NAEVUS A localised collection of pigment-forming skin cells forming a circumscribed malformation, usually brown in colour, such as a mole or a birthmark.

NEOPLASM Newgrowth. An abnormal growth of body cells. A neoplasm may be benign (usually harmless) with limited growth, or malignant, with continuous, unwanted, unlimited and uncontrolled growth (cancer).

NEPHROBLASTOMA A type of kidney cancer that occurs in infants, sometimes called Wilms' tumour.

NEUROBLASTOMA A malignant tumour of nerve-forming cells that usually arises in a special part of the nervous system called the autonomic nervous system.

NEUROMA A benign tumour composed of nerve cells.

OCCULT Concealed. Occult blood is blood which is not seen by the naked eye.

OESOPHAGUS The part of the digestive tract that allows passage of food from the mouth and pharynx to the stomach below. A muscular tube lined with epithelium extending from the neck through the chest and into the abdomen.

OESTROGEN A female sex hormone.

ONCOGENE A particular gene in a person's chromosomes that can change and become responsible for tumour-cell growth or cancer.

ONCOLOGY The study of tumours, or the study of patients suffering from tumours.

OSTEOMYELITIS Infection of bone.

PALLIATIVE Giving relief. Relieving symptoms but not curing the condition.

PANCREAS A pale fleshy gland that lies across the back of the abdominal cavity, mostly behind the stomach, responsible for secreting digestive substances into the digestive tract and insulin into the bloodstream.

PAPILLOMA A benign wart-like or fern-like tumour derived from epithelium and projecting from the epithelial lining of a surface with a central core of small blood vessels.

PET SCAN Positron emission tomography. A special technique producing 'pictures' of body tissues based on different biochemical activity in the tissues.

PHYTOESTROGENS Naturally occurring oestrogen-like hormones present in relatively large quantities in certain leguminous plants such as soybeans. Thought to be at least partly responsible for the lower incidence of some cancers (especially of the breast and the prostate) in people such as Asians who have a high intake of legumes in their diets.

PITUITARY GLAND The body's 'master gland'. A marble-sized gland in the base of the brain that controls the activity of all other glands.

PLATELETS Small disc-shaped particles in the blood that are essential for blood-clotting.

PLEURA The lining or membrane surrounding the lungs and surrounding the cavity in which the lungs move during respiration.

PLEURODESIS An artificial pleurisy created by injecting a chemical or physical irritating substance into the pleural cavity, for the purpose of causing the walls of the pleura to 'stick together', so preventing fluid from being able to collect around the lungs in the pleural cavity.

PMS Premenstrual symptoms of tension, mood changes, often depression, breast engorgement and pain and discomfort experienced a few days before menstruation.

POLYP A tumour projecting on a stalk from the mucous membrane lining the cavity of a hollow organ.

PREDNISONE A synthetic cortisone-like substance.

PROGESTERONE One of the female sex hormones.

PROSTHESIS An artificial replacement for a missing part.

PROTON-BEAM RADIOTHERAPY A new type of radiotherapy given by proton beams. The irradiation is delivered accurately and more precisely to the cancer or tumour region without affecting surrounding tissues.

RADICAL Extreme. A radical mastectomy is the surgical removal of the breast together with other nearby tissues.

RADIO-OPAQUE MATERIAL A substance that does not allow penetration of X-rays, thus showing as a white area on an X-ray film. It is commonly referred to as 'dye'. Barium and iodine are radio-opaque substances often used in X-ray studies. Lead and other metals are also radio-opaque and prevent penetration by X-rays.

RADIOTHERAPY Treatment with X-rays or gamma rays.

RESECTION Surgical removal of a part of the body.

RETICULOENDOTHELIAL SYSTEM Part of the immune system. The body system consisting of tissue defensive cells that protects the body against foreign materials and invading organisms. The special defensive cell predominantly found in bone marrow, spleen, liver and lymph nodes but also found in other tissues such as skin and soft tissues and the wall of the stomach and bowel.

SARCOMA A cancer of connective tissues such as muscle, fat, fascia or bone.

SCREENING TEST A relatively simple, safe and easily performed test that can be carried out on large numbers of people to determine whether they are likely to have a cancer or other serious disease.

SIDE EFFECT An effect other than the effect wanted.

SIGMOIDOSCOPE A long thin instrument used for passing through the anus, with a light to allow visual examination of the inside of the lower bowel.

SIGNAL HORMONE A hormone that gives a signal to stimulate activity of another hormone or cellular activity.

SPLEEN A vascular solid organ in the upper-left abdomen under the protection of the lower-left ribs. Its main function is to filter old or damaged blood cells from the bloodstream.

SQUAMOUS Squamous cells are flat scale-like cells that cover the skin, the mouth, throat, oesophagus, vagina and some other body cavities.

STEM CELL An undifferentiated precursor cell that is able to produce any type of specialised tissue cell.

STEROID   One of a group of chemical compounds with a common basic chemical structure. The naturally occurring steroids include male and female sex hormones, and hormones secreted by the cortex of the adrenal gland.

THERAPY   Treatment.

THYROXINE   A hormone produced in the thyroid gland that stimulates body activity.

TISSUE   A layer or group of cells of particular types that together perform a special function.

TOXIC   Poisonous.

TRAUMA   Injury.

TUMOUR   A swelling. The term commonly used to describe a swelling caused by a growth of cells. A newgrowth or neoplasm that may be benign (innocent) or malignant (cancer).

TUMOUR MARKER   A substance produced by a malignant tumour (cancer) that can be used to show the presence and likely size of the tumour and to indicate its response to treatment.

ULCERATIVE COLITIS   An inflammatory condition of the large bowel characterised by small ulcers in the bowel lining and causing episodes of diarrhoea.

UTERUS   The womb. The organ in the female pelvis in which a foetus develops.

VARICOSE ULCER   An ulcer in the skin, usually on the lower leg, caused by poor circulation in the tissues as a result of longstanding varicose veins.

acknowledgements

The authors wish to thank many dear patients who have become our friends. They have honoured us with their cooperation, faith and trust in their care.

We are greatly indebted to our dear wives and families for their acceptance of the long hours of absence necessary for our work.

In relation to the preparation of this book we particularly wish to thank Mavis McCarthy RN, BA (Sci), MHPE, who kindly read the manuscript and advised us how to make it more easily understandable for lay readers.

Finally we are pleased to acknowledge the cooperation of members of the Random House publishing team, especially Jill Brown and Kevin O'Brien, who had a strong commitment to making the information in this book readily available for people with cancer worries.

index